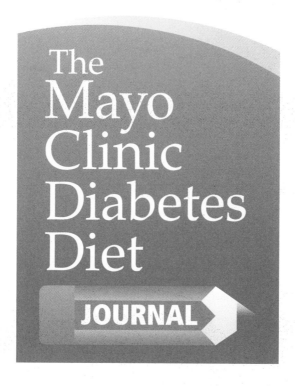

The
Mayo Clinic Diabetes Diet
JOURNAL

Good Books

Intercourse, PA 17534 • 800-762-7171 • www.GoodBooks.com

Mayo Clinic

Good Books

MEDICAL EDITOR-IN-CHIEF
Donald Hensrud, M.D.

ASSOCIATE MEDICAL EDITOR
Jennifer Nelson, R.D.

SENIOR PRODUCT MANAGER, BOOKS
Christopher Frye

DIRECTOR, HEALTH INFORMATION
Jay Maxwell

MANAGING EDITOR
Karen Wallevand

CREATIVE DIRECTOR
Daniel Brevick

ART DIRECTORS
Stewart Koski, Paul Krause,
Richard Resnick

ILLUSTRATOR
Kent McDaniel

PROOFREADERS
Miranda Attlesey, Donna Hanson

ADMINISTRATIVE ASSISTANTS
Beverly Steele,
Terri Zanto Strausbauch

Each of the habits in *Lose It!* has been the subject of scientific studies that support its role in weight management. In addition, Mayo Clinic conducted a two-week program to test the validity of this habit-based approach to quick weight loss. The 33 women who completed the program lost an average of 6.59 pounds, with individual results varying from 0.2 to 13.8 pounds lost. The 14 men who completed the program lost an average of 9.97 pounds, with individual results varying from 5.2 to 18.8 pounds lost. Individual results will vary. Consult your doctor before starting any diet program.

PUBLISHER
Merle Good

EXECUTIVE EDITOR
Phyllis Pellman Good

ASSISTANT PUBLISHER
Kate Good

Published by Good Books

© 2011 Mayo Foundation for Medical Education and Research

ISBN 978-1-56148-731-8

First Edition

If you would like more copies of this book, contact Good Books, Intercourse, PA 17534. 800-762-7171. *www.GoodBooks.com.*

For bulk sales to employers, member groups and health-related companies, contact Mayo Clinic Health Solutions, 200 First St. SW, Rochester, MN 55905, or send an email to *SpecialSalesMayoBooks@mayo.edu.*

The Mayo Clinic Diabetes Diet is intended to supplement the advice of your personal physician, whom you should consult regarding individual medical conditions. MAYO, MAYO CLINIC and the Mayo triple-shield logo are marks of Mayo Foundation for Medical Education and Research.

Photo credits: Artville, Jordan Eady and Photodisc

Cover design by Paul Krause

Printed in the USA

Table of contents

Throughout the journal you'll find this symbol, which refers you to pages in *The Mayo Clinic Diabetes Diet* book for more in-depth information.

Welcome to *The Mayo Clinic Diabetes Diet Journal* — a practical, easy-to-use resource that supports *The Mayo Clinic Diabetes Diet*

You may associate a food and activity journal with lots of busywork but very little support or follow-up.

The Mayo Clinic Diabetes Diet Journal intends to be something different. The journal guides you through the first 10 weeks of *The Mayo Clinic Diabetes Diet* in clear steps. You use simple forms to compile food and exercise records each day, as well as record your daily blood sugar (glucose) levels. In addition, the journal draws on your abilities to:

Learn from previous experience. Evaluate how you did from the previous weeks in weekly reviews and reflect on what you can do to improve your program.

Plan for the week ahead. A series of special planning tools helps you stay on track and allows you to adjust your program — based in part on what you've learned from the reviews.

These features combine to make losing weight and controlling your blood sugar more personal, pleasurable and, ultimately, more successful. What you learn about yourself during 10 weeks of journal use can carry over into a lifetime of good health.

Here's a summary of the organization and practical tools you'll find in *The Mayo Clinic Diabetes Diet Journal*.

❶ Get Started

Start the journal — and *The Mayo Clinic Diabetes Diet* — by checking your motivations for losing weight. If you feel motivated and ready, pick a start day and the weight goal you'd like to reach. You'll need to jot down some basic information to mark your starting points.

❷ Weight Record

Enter your weight from weekly weigh-ins with this tool and track how much weight you've lost from your start day. Continually update the Weight Record while using the journal.

❸ *Lose It!* Journal

This section organizes the initial two-week, quick-start portion of the diet.

Habit Tracker

Check boxes in the Tracker to follow your progress with the Add 5, Break 5 and Adopt 5 bonus habits of *Lose It!* Update the Tracker daily.

Daily Record

Record everything you eat and everything you do from day 1 through day 14 of *Lose It!* You'll also log your daily blood sugar (glucose) readings. Daily record-keeping helps keep you motivated and engaged.

Review

Assess your performance in *Lose It!* and prepare for the transition to the next stage of *The Mayo Clinic Diabetes Diet*.

❹ *Live It!* Journal

This section guides you through the next stage of *The Mayo Clinic Diabetes Diet*. Use these tools in each weekly unit for the next eight weeks:

Planner

At the beginning of each week, organize your schedule and plan ahead for upcoming activities.

Week At A Glance. Create a general overview of the coming week by scheduling meals, exercise time and other activities.

Meal Planner. Analyze meals to check how well they fit with your pyramid servings goals. Using this tool is optional but helpful.

Menu & Recipe. Refer to a sample menu each week to help guide or inspire your menu decisions.

Shopping List. Compile a list of food items to buy from the grocery store as you plan menus for the week ahead.

Daily Record

Record everything you eat and everything you do, as well as your blood sugar levels — just as you did in *Lose It!* But now, you can also include the number of pyramid servings in addition to the amounts.

Review

At the end of each week, assess your progress and review what may have worked well and what didn't work well from the previous week. Consider how to adjust and improve your program.

My motivation to lose weight

There may be many reasons why you want to lose weight. Are you physically and emotionally prepared for the effort? Take time to consider your motivations and the reasons why they matter. SEE PAGE 21 OF *THE MAYO CLINIC DIABETES DIET.*

MOTIVATION:

Why it matters:

MOTIVATION:

Why it matters:

MOTIVATION:

Why it matters:

MOTIVATION:

Why it matters:

My starting points

Are you motivated? Are your weight goals realistic? Is this a good point in your life to take on a new venture? If you can answer yes to these questions, now may be a good time to start a weight-loss program. 📖 SEE PAGE 23 OF *THE MAYO CLINIC DIABETES DIET.*

START DATE

Choose a time when you can be focused and your schedule is calm. Everyone's life includes stress, and some times are better than others to start a diet.

START WEIGHT

Be sure to weigh yourself on your start day and record the number in the box at left. Also enter your start weight in the Weight Record on page 10 of this journal.

GOAL WEIGHT

How much weight would you like to lose? Enter your goal weight in the box at left. Do you think this goal is realistic? For many people, a reasonable goal is to lose about 10 percent of their start weight. That amount is generally achievable.

BODY MASS INDEX (BMI)

The BMI takes both your weight and height into account. Refer to a BMI table and enter your BMI number in the box at left.

📖 SEE PAGE 115 OF *THE MAYO CLINIC DIABETES DIET.*

WAISTLINE MEASUREMENT

Use a flexible tape and measure around your body just above the highest points on your hipbones. Record your results in the box at left.

📖 SEE PAGE 116 OF *THE MAYO CLINIC DIABETES DIET.*

AVERAGE GLUCOSE READING

Jot down your fasting morning blood sugar (glucose) readings for three days. Take the average of those readings and record the number in the box on the left.

A1C READING

This test indicates your average blood sugar level over the past two to three months. Get your most recent reading from your doctor and record it here.

Have questions about the basics of this weight-loss program? You may find answers in *The Mayo Clinic Diabetes Diet* book.

Common questions that you may have about eating healthy, being active and losing weight are organized in the list at right. The page numbers accompanying each question cross-reference material in *The Mayo Clinic Diabetes Diet* book that may provide you with answers.

Basics

What is the Mayo Clinic Healthy Weight Pyramid?	130-143
What is my healthy weight?	112-119
What is my daily calorie goal?	77
What are my daily serving recommendations?	79
How much is in a serving?	81

Healthy eating

How do I create a weekly menu?	82-87
What are healthy shopping strategies?	170-172
What are the serving sizes of different foods?	222-249
How do I overcome barriers to healthy eating?	192-221

Activity and exercise

How do I start exercising?	38-39, 58-59
How many calories do I burn when I'm active?	191
How do I increase the amount of activity I do?	104, 184-191
How do I set up a good exercise program?	101-105

Behaviors

How do I set goals?	74-76
How do I change a behavior?	144-153
How can I stay motivated?	161
What can I do when I slip up?	154-167

THE BEST WAY TO WEIGH IN

With *The Mayo Clinic Diabetes Diet*, you'll weigh yourself at least once a week. Record the results in your Weight Record.

How regularly should you weigh yourself? That depends. Checking the scale too often can cause you to obsess over minor daily weight changes. Not checking enough may indicate that you're not focused and involved with your weight program.

A good rule of thumb is to weigh yourself about once a week. If you feel a need to do so more often — several times a week or even daily — that's OK. Just remember that the long-term weight trends occurring over weeks or months are generally more important to know than are day-to-day changes.

Be consistent with your weigh-ins from week to week. Schedule them on a regular day and at a regular time and try to stick with that routine. Along with providing more uniform results in your Weight Record, consistency also helps to keep you engaged in your weight-loss program.

You'll need to weigh yourself on your start day of *The Mayo Clinic Diabetes Diet*. It's important that you enter your start weight at two places in the journal:

✔ Weight Record (page 10)

✔ Day 1 of the Daily Record (page 18)

Later, you'll be reminded on the seventh day of each week to weigh yourself and record the weight in your Daily Record. You'll also continue to update and chart your progress in the Weight Record.

Use weigh-ins to review your progress. Be sure to reward yourself when you meet your weight goals. If you don't meet your goals, don't be too hard on yourself. Identify factors that may have worked against you and consider how to avoid them.

Weight Record

 START WEIGHT:

End of week weigh-in (write your weight in the boxes below)

| 1 | 2 | 3 | 4 | 5 | 6 | 7 | 8 | 9 | 10 |

Weight change (in pounds)

+4
+3
+2
+1
0
-1
-2
-3
-4
-5
-6
-7
-8
-9
-10
-11
-12
-13
-14
-15
-16
-17
-18
-19
-20
-21
-22
-23
-24
-25
-26
-27
-28
-29
-30

Lose It!   Live It!

	11	12	13	14	15	16

Weight change (in pounds)

+4
+3
+2
+1
0
-1
-2
-3
-4
-5
-6
-7
-8
-9
-10
-11
-12
-13
-14
-15
-16
-17
-18
-19
-20
-21
-22
-23
-24
-25
-26
-27
-28
-29
-30

Bonus weeks

DIRECTIONS:

1. Write your start weight in the box at the top of the page.

2. After each weekly weigh-in, write your current weight in the box under the appropriate week.

3. Subtract your current weight from your start weight to calculate your weight change.

4. Mark your weight change for each week on the table.

5. Connect the marks to form a line graph of your progress.

Lose It!

This section of *The Mayo Clinic Diabetes Diet Journal* is designed to help you safely lose weight over a two-week period to jump-start your weight loss efforts. During this time, you'll also monitor your blood sugar (glucose). It's easy to get started.

How to record *Lose It!*

❶ Start each day by setting a realistic, achievable goal in the Daily Record.

❷ Record the amount of time you spend doing exercise and being active. The activity should be moderately intense and sustained for five minutes or more.

❸ Record everything you eat during the day, including amounts (in most cases, your best estimate will do).

❹ Record your blood sugar (glucose) level twice daily: your a.m. fasting reading and your p.m. reading before dinner. How often you need to test your blood sugar is very individual. Go by your doctor's recommendations.

❺ At the end of each day, mark the Habit Tracker to indicate which of the Add 5, Break 5 and Bonus 5 habits you successfully achieved.

❻ Following day 7 and day 14, total the rows and columns of the Habit Tracker. This may help you identify problems and improve your program.

❼ Following day 14, use the Review to assess your progress in *Lose It!* and prepare for your switch to *Live It!*

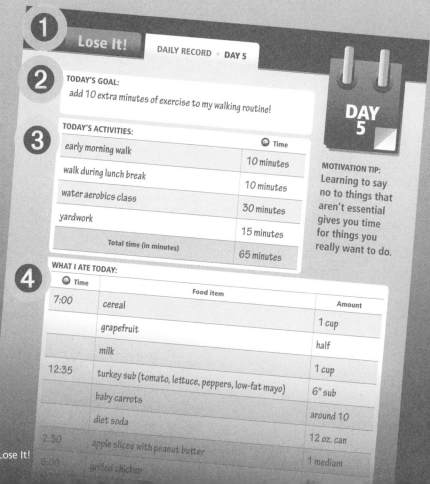

Lose It!   DAILY RECORD · DAY 5

TODAY'S GOAL:
add 10 extra minutes of exercise to my walking routine!

DAY 5

TODAY'S ACTIVITIES:

	Time
early morning walk	10 minutes
walk during lunch break	10 minutes
water aerobics class	30 minutes
yardwork	15 minutes
Total time (in minutes)	65 minutes

MOTIVATION TIP:
Learning to say no to things that aren't essential gives you time for things you really want to do.

WHAT I ATE TODAY:

Time	Food item	Amount
7:00	cereal	1 cup
	grapefruit	half
	milk	1 cup
12:35	turkey sub (tomato, lettuce, peppers, low-fat mayo)	6" sub
	baby carrots	around 10
	diet soda	12 oz. can
2:30	apple slices with peanut butter	1 medium
6:00	grilled chicken	

WEEK 1 HABIT TRACKER

✓ Check if done	Day 1	Day 2	Day 3	Day 4	Day 5	Day 6	Day 7	TOTALS
ADD 5 HABITS				✓		✓	✓	5
1. Eat a healthy breakfast	✓	✓			✓		✓	5
2. Eat vegetables and fruits	✓	✓	✓			✓	✓	5
3. Eat whole grains	✓	✓	✓		✓		✓	6
4. Eat healthy fats	✓	✓	✓	✓	✓	✓	✓	5
5. Move!	✓				✓	✓	✓	5
BREAK 5 HABITS						✓		✓	3
1. No TV while eating				✓		✓	✓	6
2. No sugar	✓	✓	✓					

My start weight	185
Minus my weight today	177
= Equals my weight change	8

I FEEL:
- ☑ Terrific
- ○ Good
- ○ So-so
- ○ Discouraged
- ○ Like giving up

THE RESULTS FROM *LOSE IT!*:
- ○ Far exceeded my expectations
- ☑ Were better than I expected
- ○ Met my expectations
- ○ Were not as good as I expected
- ○ Fell far short of my expectations

ASSESSING YOUR HABIT TRACKER:

Days

	1	2	3	4	5	6	7	8	9	10	11	12	13	14
15														
14														
13														

WEEK 1 HABIT TRACKER								
✓ Check if done	Day 1	Day 2	Day 3	Day 4	Day 5	Day 6	Day 7	TOTALS
ADD 5 HABITS								
1. Eat a healthy breakfast								
2. Eat vegetables and fruits								
3. Eat whole grains								
4. Eat healthy fats								
5. Move!								
BREAK 5 HABITS								
1. No TV while eating								
2. No sugar								
3. No snacks								
4. Only moderate meat and dairy								
5. No eating at restaurants								
5 BONUS HABITS								
1. Keep diet records								
2. Keep exercise/activity records								
3. Move more!								
4. Eat "real" food								
5. Write your daily goals								
Totals								

DIRECTIONS:
1. At the end of each day, check off which Add, Break and Bonus habits you have completed.
2. At the end of the week, total the columns and the rows to see how you've progressed.

WEEK 2 HABIT TRACKER							
Day 8	Day 9	Day 10	Day 11	Day 12	Day 13	Day 14	TOTALS
ADD 5 HABITS							
BREAK 5 HABITS							
5 BONUS HABITS							

REMINDER:

Total the columns and rows of your Habit Tracker to see which habits you're having success with and which are a problem for you.

See pages 66-67 of *The Mayo Clinic Diabetes Diet.*

The sample above demonstrates how to fill out your Habit Tracker.

DAY 1

TODAY'S GOAL:

TODAY'S ACTIVITIES: 🕐 Time

Total time (in minutes)	

MY START WEIGHT:

WHAT I ATE TODAY:

🕐 Time	Food item	Amount

GLUCOSE READINGS:

A.M. fasting	P.M. before dinner

DAY 2

TODAY'S GOAL:

TODAY'S ACTIVITIES: ⏱ Time

Total time (in minutes)	

MOTIVATION TIP:
Write down all the benefits of losing weight. Rank your top three reasons. Refer to the list frequently.

WHAT I ATE TODAY:

⏱ Time	Food item	Amount

GLUCOSE READINGS:

A.M. fasting	P.M. before dinner

DAY 3

TODAY'S GOAL:

TODAY'S ACTIVITIES: 🕐 Time

Total time (in minutes)	

MOTIVATION TIP:
It takes time for the healthy new behaviors you're learning to become habits. Every step, every day, is important.

WHAT I ATE TODAY:

🕐 Time	Food item	Amount

GLUCOSE READINGS:

A.M. fasting	P.M. before dinner

DAY 4

TODAY'S GOAL:

TODAY'S ACTIVITIES:

🕐 Time

Total time (in minutes)	

MOTIVATION TIP:

Getting support from others is not a sign of weakness. If you feel that you need help, ask for it.

WHAT I ATE TODAY:

🕐 Time	Food item	Amount

GLUCOSE READINGS:

A.M. fasting	P.M. before dinner

DAY 5

TODAY'S GOAL:

TODAY'S ACTIVITIES: 🕐 **Time**

Total time (in minutes)	

MOTIVATION TIP:
Learning to say no to things that aren't essential gives you time for things you really want to do.

WHAT I ATE TODAY:

🕐 Time	Food item	Amount

GLUCOSE READINGS:

A.M. fasting	P.M. before dinner

DAY 6

TODAY'S GOAL:

TODAY'S ACTIVITIES: 🕐 Time

Total time (in minutes)	

MOTIVATION TIP:

Check restaurant Web sites for menus. You can look for healthy options before you eat there.

WHAT I ATE TODAY:

🕐 Time	Food item	Amount

GLUCOSE READINGS:

A.M. fasting	P.M. before dinner

DAY 7

TODAY'S GOAL:

TODAY'S ACTIVITIES: ⏱ Time

Total time (in minutes)	

MY WEIGHT TODAY:

WHAT I ATE TODAY:

⏱ Time	Food item	Amount

GLUCOSE READINGS:

A.M. fasting	P.M. before dinner

DAY 8

TODAY'S GOAL:

TODAY'S ACTIVITIES: ⏱ Time

Total time (in minutes)	

MOTIVATION TIP:

Change your exercise routine occasionally and do a variety of activities to avoid workout boredom.

WHAT I ATE TODAY:

⏱ Time	Food item	Amount

GLUCOSE READINGS:

A.M. fasting	P.M. before dinner

DAY 9

TODAY'S GOAL:

TODAY'S ACTIVITIES: Time

Total time (in minutes)	

MOTIVATION TIP:

Don't think too far ahead. Look at what you can do today to make your program work for you.

WHAT I ATE TODAY:

Time	Food item	Amount

GLUCOSE READINGS:

A.M. fasting	P.M. before dinner

DAY 10

TODAY'S GOAL:

TODAY'S ACTIVITIES: ⏱ Time

Total time (in minutes)	

MOTIVATION TIP:

Reward yourself with something that matters to you every time you reach a goal.

WHAT I ATE TODAY:

⏱ Time	Food item	Amount

GLUCOSE READINGS:

A.M. fasting	P.M. before dinner

DAY 11

TODAY'S GOAL:

TODAY'S ACTIVITIES: 🕐 Time

Total time (in minutes)	

MOTIVATION TIP:
Choose exercises that you can do regardless of the weather, such as mall walking or indoor swimming.

WHAT I ATE TODAY:

🕐 Time	Food item	Amount

GLUCOSE READINGS:

A.M. fasting	P.M. before dinner

TODAY'S GOAL:

TODAY'S ACTIVITIES:

	⏱ Time
Total time (in minutes)	

WHAT I ATE TODAY:

⏱ Time	Food item	Amount

GLUCOSE READINGS:

A.M. fasting	P.M. before dinner

DAY 13

TODAY'S GOAL:

TODAY'S ACTIVITIES: 🕐 Time

Total time (in minutes)	

MOTIVATION TIP:
Negative self-talk can produce anxiety. Be aware of what you say to yourself and try to make it more positive.

WHAT I ATE TODAY:

🕐 Time	Food item	Amount

GLUCOSE READINGS:

A.M. fasting	P.M. before dinner

DAY 14

TODAY'S GOAL:

TODAY'S ACTIVITIES:

⏱ **Time**

Total time (in minutes)	

MY WEIGHT TODAY:

WHAT I ATE TODAY:

⏱ Time	Food item	Amount

GLUCOSE READINGS:

A.M. fasting	P.M. before dinner

My start weight [ ]

Minus my weight today [ ]

= Equals my weight change [ ]

I FEEL:
- Terrific
- Good
- So-so
- Discouraged
- Like giving up

THE RESULTS FROM *LOSE IT!*:
- Far exceeded my expectations
- Were better than I expected
- Met my expectations
- Were not as good as I expected
- Fell far short of my expectations

ASSESSING YOUR HABIT TRACKER:

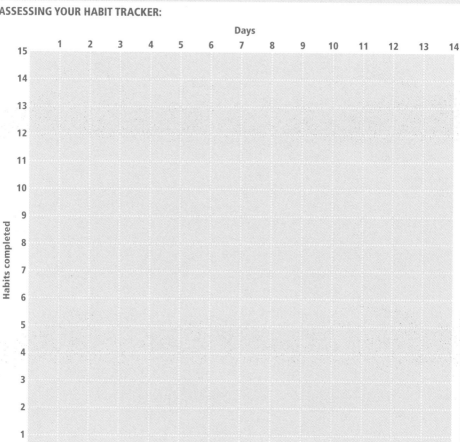

Days

(Habits completed)

DIRECTIONS:

For each day of *Lose It!*, mark a dot on the graph to indicate the number of check marks you entered in your Habit Tracker. Then connect the dots to show the entire 14 days.

See a sample chart on the next page ➔

NOTE:

On some days you'll have fewer check marks than on other days — that's to be expected. But on most days, consider 10 check marks to be a reasonable mark of success. The days when you have more than 10 check marks are all the better!

WHICH HABITS WERE STRENGTHS FOR YOU? CAN YOU LIST REASONS WHY YOU DID WELL?

HOW MOTIVATED ARE YOU TO TRANSITION INTO *LIVE IT!*?
- Extremely
- Confident
- Somewhat
- Not very
- Not at all

See page 69 of *The Mayo Clinic Diabetes Diet.*

WHICH HABITS DID YOU FIND MOST CHALLENGING? WHY WERE THEY MORE DIFFICULT?

CAN YOU SEE TRENDS IN YOUR BLOOD SUGAR (GLUCOSE) LEVELS?
(For example, are the numbers are getting lower or becoming more consistent?)

ASSESSING YOUR HABIT TRACKER:

CAN YOU IDENTIFY STRATEGIES TO HELP YOU AVOID CHALLENGING OR DISRUPTIVE SITUATIONS?

The sample above shows how you can fill out your Habit Tracker assessment.

Live It!

This section of *The Mayo Clinic Diabetes Diet Journal* is designed to help you continue losing weight — about 1 to 2 pounds a week — until you reach your goal weight, and then to maintain that weight as you *Live It!* for the rest of your life.

How to plan *Live It!*

Start each week with the Planner, which can help organize your week and guide your food and exercise decisions.

❶ Use the Week At A Glance to create an overview of your meals, exercise and activity schedule, and events and special plans for the week ahead.

❷ The Meal Planner allows you to check how well a meal fits in your daily recommended servings goals. This is an optional feature that you may choose for one or two meals during the week.

❸ Add items to the Shopping List as you plan your daily menus. That will help you save time and money on your next shopping trip.

Continue to monitor your blood sugar (glucose) level as recommended by your doctor. Keep in mind that because your weight may not change as quickly during this period, the changes in your blood sugar may not be as noticeable. They may be more gradual.

❶ Live It!

WEEK 2 PLANNER • WEEK AT A GLANCE

Day	Breakfast	Lunch	Dinner	Snack
EXAMPLE	cereal banana	spaghetti fruit salad	tuna wrap baby carrots	crackers and cheese
1	blueberry pancake milk	dilled pasta salad apple	rosemary chicken baked potato cauliflower	cherry tomatoes
2	toast & jam grapefruit	California burger pear	Greek salad crackers	baby carrots & dip
3	fruit yogurt parfait small muffin	turkey sandwich mixed greens with dressing	pasta primavera apple	celery & peanut butter
4	muffins pear halves	chicken wrap sliced tomato	beef kebabs potatoes pineapple ring	mixed berries
5	English muffin grapefruit	Southwestern salad pita bread	spaghetti with tomato sauce zucchini	peanuts
6	hard-boiled egg toast	pita bread with hummus	grilled fish	cherry

MAIN MEAL OR MEALS OF THE DAY	HOW MUCH
Dinner	
grilled chicken breast	2 1/2 oz
baby potatoes	3
steamed broccoli	2 cups
margarine	1 tsp
pear	1 small

EASY AS 1, 2, 3:
This page allows
you to check
how well a meal
meets your
recommended
servings goals.

❶ Write down what
you're planning to eat
for this meal (or to...

③ Live It! WEEK 2 PLANNER · SHOPPING LIST

Fresh produce	Whole grains	Meat & dairy
10 large tomatoes	8 oz. package spaghetti	salmon fillets
2 red peppers	1 loaf rye bread	chicken breasts
summer squash	1 package English muffins	milk
zucchini	bag of pita bread	yogurt
1 bag baby carrots		
cherries		
3 grapefruit		

PLAN AHEAD:
Create your
Shopping List
the week bef
going to the
grocery stor
You'll have a
the ingredie
on hand at t
time you ji...

How to record *Live It!*

❶ Start each day by setting a realistic, achievable goal in the Daily Record.

❷ Record everything you eat, including amounts and the number of pyramid servings.

❸ Record how much time you spend doing exercise and being active. Activity should be moderately intense and sustained for five minutes or more.

❹ Following day 7, take time to assess your progress in the weekly Review.

Live It!   WEEK 2 ▪ **REVIEW**   Re-examine how your week went.

| My start weight | | I FEEL: ● Terrific ● Good | I'M MOST PROUD OF: |

Minus my

Live It!   WEEK 2 DAILY RECORD ▪ **DAY 6**

TODAY'S DATE: Saturday 7/19

1

TODAY'S GOAL:
will eat at home today ~ no eating out!

NOTES ABOUT TODAY:
need to get my walk in before breakfast ~ Alex has a game @ 4:30pm

2

WHAT I ATE TODAY:

Number of servings per food group

⏱ Time	Food item	Amount	V	F	C	PD	Ft	S
7:30	bagel	1			2			1
"	raspberry jam	1 1/2 tbsp						
"	banana	1		1				
"	skim milk	1 cup				1		
12:10	vegetable soup	1 cup	1					
"	lettuce salad w/dressing	2 cups	1					1
	yogurt w/berries							

NEW FOOD I WOULD LIKE TO TRY:

WEEK 2
DAY 6

TODAY'S ACTIVITIES:	🕐 Time
early morning walk	30 minutes
mow the lawn ③	45 minutes
walk to the ballgame	15 minutes
Total time (in minutes)	90 minutes

MOTIVATION TIP:
Different fruits provide different nutrients, so variety is vital to get all the health benefits. Use them for snacks and at every meal.

KEY:
- **V** Vegetables
- **F** Fruits
- **C** Carbohydrates
- **PD** Protein/Dairy
- **Ft** Fats
- **S** Sweets

Sweets
75 calories a day or 525 calories a week
75 ← Write in your calories here.

Fats ✗ ✗

Protein/Dairy ✗ ✗ ✗

Carbohydrates ✗ ✗ ✗ ✗

Day	Breakfast	Lunch	Dinner	Snack
EXAMPLE	cereal banana	spaghetti fruit salad	tuna wrap baby carrots	crackers and cheese
1				
2				
3				
4				
5				
6				
7				

Exercise and activities	Events and special plans
swim class @ 11am walk to work	kids ballgame @ 6pm note: supper will be on the go

WEEK AT A GLANCE

USING THE PLANNER:

Organize your plans for meals, activities and exercise in the coming week. Note upcoming events that may affect your weight program, such as travel, eating out, social occasions and vacations.

MAIN MEAL OR MEALS OF THE DAY	HOW MUCH

EASY AS 1, 2, 3:

This page allows you to check how well a meal meets your recommended servings goals.

1. Write down what you're planning to eat for this meal (or for the entire day).

2. Calculate the number of servings based on how much you're planning to eat.

3. Be sure to include the food items from your menu in your Shopping List.

PYRAMID SERVINGS FOR THIS MEAL

Sweets (in calories)		
Fats		
Protein/Dairy		
Carbohydrates		
Fruits & Vegetables	Fruits	Vegetables

◀ Check off the number of servings on the pyramid at left.

MAIN MEAL OR MEALS OF THE DAY	HOW MUCH

EASY AS 1, 2, 3:

This page allows you to check how well a meal meets your recommended servings goals.

1. Write down what you're planning to eat for this meal (or for the entire day).

2. Calculate the number of servings based on how much you're planning to eat.

3. Be sure to include the food items from your menu in your Shopping List.

PYRAMID SERVINGS FOR THIS MEAL

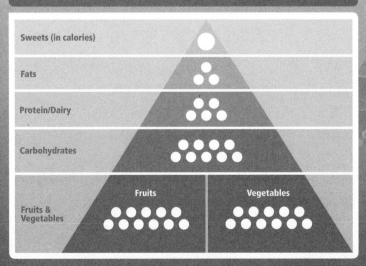

Sweets (in calories)

Fats

Protein/Dairy

Carbohydrates

Fruits

Vegetables

Fruits & Vegetables

◀ Check off the number of servings on the pyramid at left.

MENU FOR THE DAY

BREAKFAST

1 medium hard-boiled egg
1 slice whole-grain toast
1 tsp. trans fat-free margarine
1 medium orange
Calorie-free beverage

V	F	C	PD	Ft	S
0	1	1	1	1	0

LUNCH

Open-faced roast beef sandwich
*8 cherry tomatoes
1 small apple
Calorie-free beverage

V	F	C	PD	Ft	S
1	1	1	1	0	0

DINNER

1 serving Pasta with Marinara Sauce
  and Grilled Vegetables
¾ c. blueberries with ¼ c. nondairy
  whipped topping
Calorie-free beverage

V	F	C	PD	Ft	S
3	1	2	0	2	0

SNACK

1 c. fat-free, reduced-calorie yogurt

V	F	C	PD	Ft	S
0	0	0	1	0	0

*The serving size stated is the minimum
amount. Eat as much as you wish.

QUICK TIP:

The menu on this page demonstrates how you can plan your own daily menus. Feel free to include this sample on one of your days.

DINNER RECIPE

Pasta With Marinara Sauce and Grilled Vegetables (SERVES 8)

2 tbsp. olive oil
10 large fresh tomatoes, peeled
   and diced
1 tsp. salt
½ tsp. minced garlic
2 tbsp. chopped onion
1 tsp. dried basil
1 tsp. sugar
½ tsp. oregano
   Black pepper, to taste
2 red peppers, sliced into chunks
1 yellow summer squash, sliced
   lengthwise
1 zucchini, sliced lengthwise
1 sweet onion, sliced into ¼-inch
   rounds
1 12-oz. package of whole-wheat
   spaghetti

- Heat oil in a heavy skillet. Add tomatoes, salt, garlic, onions, basil, sugar, oregano and black pepper. Cook slowly, uncovered, for 30 minutes or until sauce is thickened.

- Brush peppers, squash, zucchini and onion with oil. Place under broiler and cook, turning frequently until browned and tender. Remove to bowl.

- Cook spaghetti until al dente. Drain well and portion onto plates. Cover with equal amounts of sauce. Top with equal amounts of vegetables. Serve immediately.

Fresh produce	Whole grains	Meat & dairy

Frozen goods	Canned goods	Miscellaneous

WEEK 1 PLANNER

SHOPPING LIST

QUICK TIP:

Create your shopping list for the week before going to the grocery store. You'll have all the ingredients on hand at the time you prepare a meal.

Fresh produce	Whole grains
10 large tomatoes	8 oz package spaghetti
2 red peppers	1 loaf rye brea
summer squash	1 package English muffir
zucchini	
1 bag baby carrots	bag of pita
cherries	
3 grapefruit	

▲
Add to your Shopping List as you plan your menus for the week.

TODAY'S DATE:

TODAY'S GOAL:

NOTES ABOUT TODAY:

WHAT I ATE TODAY: Number of servings per food group

Time	Food item	Amount	V	F	C	PD	Ft	S

GLUCOSE READINGS:

A.M. fasting	P.M. before dinner

TODAY'S ACTIVITIES: 🕑 **Time**

Total time (in minutes)	

MOTIVATION TIP:
Don't worry too much about recording the exact number of servings of vegetables and fruits. You can eat, within reason, unlimited amounts of vegetables and generous amounts of fruit.

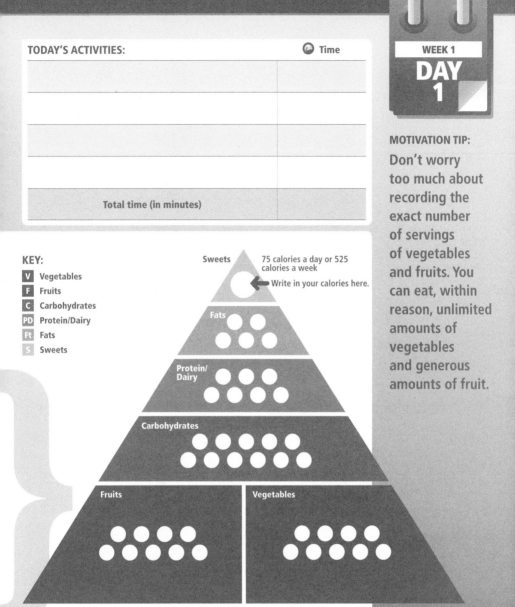

KEY:

- **V** Vegetables
- **F** Fruits
- **C** Carbohydrates
- **PD** Protein/Dairy
- **Ft** Fats
- **S** Sweets

Sweets — 75 calories a day or 525 calories a week
◄ Write in your calories here.

Fats

Protein/Dairy

Carbohydrates

Fruits

Vegetables

WHAT I ATE TODAY FROM THE PYRAMID:
Check off the circles in the food group servings above as you record food and beverage items in the table at left. For sweets, give your best estimate of the total number of calories for the day.

TODAY'S DATE:

TODAY'S GOAL:

NOTES ABOUT TODAY:

WHAT I ATE TODAY:　　　　　　　　　　　　　Number of servings per food group

🕐 Time	Food item	Amount	V	F	C	PD	Ft	S

GLUCOSE READINGS:

A.M. fasting	P.M. before dinner

TODAY'S ACTIVITIES:

🕐 Time

Total time (in minutes)	

WEEK 1

DAY 2

MOTIVATION TIP:

A common mistake is to start off exercising too much and too hard. If your body isn't used to this exertion, your muscles may feel stiff and sore, causing you to exercise less or skip it altogether.

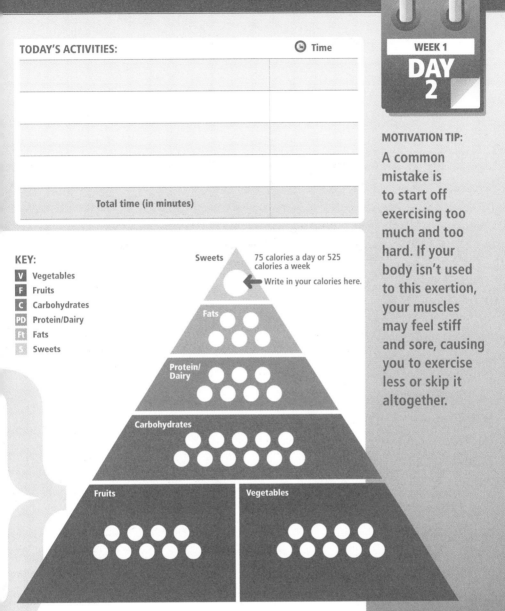

KEY:

- **V** Vegetables
- **F** Fruits
- **C** Carbohydrates
- **PD** Protein/Dairy
- **Ft** Fats
- **S** Sweets

Sweets

75 calories a day or 525 calories a week

← Write in your calories here.

Fats

Protein/Dairy

Carbohydrates

Fruits

Vegetables

WHAT I ATE TODAY FROM THE PYRAMID:

Check off the circles in the food group servings above as you record food and beverage items in the table at left. For sweets, give your best estimate of the total number of calories for the day.

TODAY'S DATE:

TODAY'S GOAL:

NOTES ABOUT TODAY:

WHAT I ATE TODAY: Number of servings per food group

Time	Food item	Amount	V	F	C	PD	Ft	S

GLUCOSE READINGS:

A.M. fasting	P.M. before dinner

TODAY'S ACTIVITIES:

🕐 **Time**

Total time (in minutes)	

MOTIVATION TIP:
Friends — even spouses — may sometimes feel intimidated by your efforts to lose weight. It's up to you to let them know how important their support is to you.

KEY:

- **V** Vegetables
- **F** Fruits
- **C** Carbohydrates
- **PD** Protein/Dairy
- **Ft** Fats
- **S** Sweets

Sweets — 75 calories a day or 525 calories a week
← Write in your calories here.

Fats

Protein/Dairy

Carbohydrates

Fruits

Vegetables

WHAT I ATE TODAY FROM THE PYRAMID:
Check off the circles in the food group servings above as you record food and beverage items in the table at left. For sweets, give your best estimate of the total number of calories for the day.

TODAY'S DATE:

TODAY'S GOAL:

NOTES ABOUT TODAY:

WHAT I ATE TODAY: Number of servings per food group

Time	Food item	Amount	V	F	C	PD	Ft	S

GLUCOSE READINGS:

A.M. fasting	P.M. before dinner

TODAY'S ACTIVITIES: 🕐 **Time**

Total time (in minutes)	

MOTIVATION TIP:

When you know you'll be eating out (and eating extra calories), try to increase the amount of exercise you do on that day.

KEY:

V Vegetables
F Fruits
C Carbohydrates
PD Protein/Dairy
Ft Fats
S Sweets

Sweets   75 calories a day or 525 calories a week
← Write in your calories here.

Fats

Protein/ Dairy

Carbohydrates

Fruits   **Vegetables**

WHAT I ATE TODAY FROM THE PYRAMID:

Check off the circles in the food group servings above as you record food and beverage items in the table at left. For sweets, give your best estimate of the total number of calories for the day.

TODAY'S DATE:

TODAY'S GOAL:

NOTES ABOUT TODAY:

WHAT I ATE TODAY: Number of servings per food group

⏱ Time	Food item	Amount	V	F	C	PD	Ft	S

GLUCOSE READINGS:

A.M. fasting	P.M. before dinner

TODAY'S ACTIVITIES:

🕐 **Time**

Total time (in minutes)	

MOTIVATION TIP:
Choose activities that fit your personality. If you prefer solitude, consider walking or jogging. If group activities appeal to you, consider an aerobics class or golf league.

KEY:

- **V** Vegetables
- **F** Fruits
- **C** Carbohydrates
- **PD** Protein/Dairy
- **Ft** Fats
- **S** Sweets

Sweets

75 calories a day or 525 calories a week

Write in your calories here.

Fats

Protein/Dairy

Carbohydrates

Fruits

Vegetables

WHAT I ATE TODAY FROM THE PYRAMID:
Check off the circles in the food group servings above as you record food and beverage items in the table at left. For sweets, give your best estimate of the total number of calories for the day.

TODAY'S DATE:

TODAY'S GOAL:

NOTES ABOUT TODAY:

WHAT I ATE TODAY: Number of servings per food group

🕐 Time	Food item	Amount	V	F	C	PD	Ft	S

GLUCOSE READINGS:

A.M. fasting	P.M. before dinner

TODAY'S ACTIVITIES:

🕐 **Time**

Total time (in minutes)	

MOTIVATION TIP:
Learn to recognize true hunger and ignore cravings. If you ate just a couple of hours ago and your stomach isn't rumbling, give the craving time to pass before you reach for a snack. Be sure the snack fits your meal plan.

KEY:

V	Vegetables
F	Fruits
C	Carbohydrates
PD	Protein/Dairy
Ft	Fats
S	Sweets

Sweets

75 calories a day or 525 calories a week

← Write in your calories here.

Fats

Protein/Dairy

Carbohydrates

Fruits

Vegetables

WHAT I ATE TODAY FROM THE PYRAMID:
Check off the circles in the food group servings above as you record food and beverage items in the table at left. For sweets, give your best estimate of the total number of calories for the day.

TODAY'S DATE:

TODAY'S GOAL:

NOTES ABOUT TODAY:
It's weigh-in day ~ record my weight in the weekly Review and the Weight Record.

WHAT I ATE TODAY: Number of servings per food group

Time	Food item	Amount	V	F	C	PD	Ft	S

GLUCOSE READINGS:

A.M. fasting	P.M. before dinner

TODAY'S ACTIVITIES:

🕐 **Time**

Total time (in minutes)	

REMINDER:

Record your weight for today in the weekly Review and the Weight Record.

KEY:

- **V** Vegetables
- **F** Fruits
- **C** Carbohydrates
- **PD** Protein/Dairy
- **Ft** Fats
- **S** Sweets

Sweets — 75 calories a day or 525 calories a week

← Write in your calories here.

Fats

Protein/Dairy

Carbohydrates

Fruits

Vegetables

WHAT I ATE TODAY FROM THE PYRAMID:

Check off the circles in the food group servings above as you record food and beverage items in the table at left. For sweets, give your best estimate of the total number of calories for the day.

My start weight

Minus my weight today

= Equals my weight change

I FEEL:
- Terrific
- Good
- So-so
- Discouraged
- Like giving up

I'M MOST PROUD OF:

WHAT WORKED WELL:

WHAT DIDN'T WORK AS WELL:

DID I REACH MY SERVINGS GOALS FOR THIS WEEK?

Food group	Daily servings	Day 1	Day 2	Day 3	Day 4	Day 5	Day 6	Day 7
Vegetables		○	○	○	○	○	○	○
Fruits		○	○	○	○	○	○	○
Carbohydrates		○	○	○	○	○	○	○
Protein/Dairy		○	○	○	○	○	○	○
Fats		○	○	○	○	○	○	○
Sweets		○	○	○	○	○	○	○

DIRECTIONS:
1. Write your daily serving goals for each food group in the table above.
2. Compare the serving totals that you recorded for each day of the past week with your goals.
3. Check off the circles in the table above if your serving totals have met your goals.

CHANGES IN MY BLOOD SUGAR (GLUCOSE) READINGS:

REMINDER: Calculate your weight change in this Review and record it in the Weight Record.

NEW FOODS OR ACTIVITIES I WOULD LIKE TO TRY:

HOW MANY STEPS A DAY DID I TAKE (IF I USED A PEDOMETER)?

Day 1	Day 2	Day 3	Day 4	Day 5	Day 6	Day 7

HOW MANY MINUTES A DAY WAS I ACTIVE?

DID I REACH MY SERVINGS GOALS FOR THIS W

Food group	Daily servings	Day 1	Da
Vegetables	4+	✓	
Fruits	3+		✓
Carbohydrates	4	✓	✓
Protein/Dairy	3	✓	✓
Fats	3		✓

DIRECTIONS:

1. Add a dot for your total minutes of activity for each day of last week.
2. Connect each dot on the chart with a line.

See a sample chart to the right. →

The samples above show how you can fill out your servings goals table and your activity chart for your weekly Review.

Day	Breakfast	Lunch	Dinner	Snack
EXAMPLE	cereal banana	spaghetti fruit salad	tuna wrap baby carrots	crackers and cheese
1				
2				
3				
4				
5				
6				
7				

Exercise and activities	Events and special plans
swim class @ 11am walk to work	kids ballgame @ 6pm note: supper will be on the go

USING THE PLANNER:

Organize your plans for meals, activities and exercise in the coming week. Note upcoming events that may affect your weight program, such as travel, eating out, social occasions and vacations.

WEEK 2 PLANNER
MEAL PLANNER

MAIN MEAL OR MEALS OF THE DAY	HOW MUCH

EASY AS 1, 2, 3:

This page allows you to check how well a meal meets your recommended servings goals.

1. Write down what you're planning to eat for this meal (or for the entire day).

2. Calculate the number of servings based on how much you're planning to eat.

3. Be sure to include the food items from your menu in your Shopping List.

PYRAMID SERVINGS FOR THIS MEAL

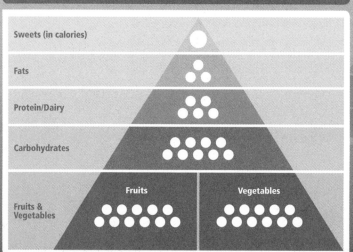

Sweets (in calories)

Fats

Protein/Dairy

Carbohydrates

Fruits

Vegetables

Fruits & Vegetables

◀ Check off the number of servings on the pyramid at left.

MAIN MEAL OR MEALS OF THE DAY	HOW MUCH

EASY AS 1, 2, 3:

This page allows you to check how well a meal meets your recommended servings goals.

1. Write down what you're planning to eat for this meal (or for the entire day).
2. Calculate the number of servings based on how much you're planning to eat.
3. Be sure to include the food items from your menu in your Shopping List.

PYRAMID SERVINGS FOR THIS MEAL

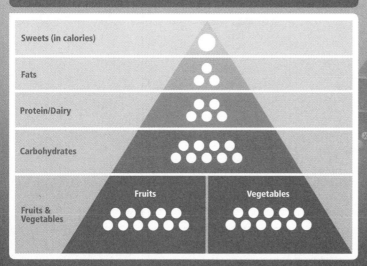

Sweets (in calories)

Fats

Protein/Dairy

Carbohydrates

Fruits   Vegetables

Fruits & Vegetables

75

◄ Check off the number of servings on the pyramid at left.

Live It!

MENU FOR THE DAY

BREAKFAST
1 pancake (4-inch diameter)
¾ c. blueberries or other berries
1 tsp. trans fat-free margarine
1½ tbsp. syrup
1 c. skim milk
Calorie-free beverage

V	F	C	PD	Ft	S
0	1	1	1	1	0

LUNCH
1 serving Dilled Pasta Salad With
   Spring Vegetables
1 small apple
Calorie-free beverage

V	F	C	PD	Ft	S
1	1	2	0	1	0

DINNER
1 serving Rosemary Chicken
⅓ c. brown rice mixed with ½ cup
   chopped green onion
*1½ c. green beans
1 medium orange
Calorie-free beverage

V	F	C	PD	Ft	S
3	1	1	2	1	0

SNACK
*1 serving favorite fruit

V	F	C	PD	Ft	S
0	1	0	0	0	0

*The serving size stated is the minimum
amount. Eat as much as you wish.

QUICK TIP:

The menu on this page demonstrates how you can plan your own daily menus. Feel free to include this sample on one of your days.

LUNCH RECIPE

Dilled Pasta Salad With Spring Vegetables (SERVES 8)

3 c. shell pasta (medium-sized)
8 asparagus spears, cut into ½-inch
    pieces
1 c. halved cherry tomatoes
1 c. sliced green peppers
½ c. chopped green onions

FOR THE DRESSING:

¼ c. olive oil
2 tbsp. lemon juice
2 tbsp. rice or white wine vinegar
2 tsp. dill weed
Cracked black pepper, to taste

- Cook and drain pasta. Rinse in cold water. Put into a bowl.

- In a saucepan, cover asparagus with water. Cook until tender-crisp, 3 to 5 minutes. Drain and rinse with cold water. Add asparagus, tomatoes, green peppers and onions to pasta.

- In a small bowl, whisk together the ingredients for the dressing. Pour dressing over the pasta and vegetables. Toss to coat. Cover, refrigerate and serve.

DINNER RECIPE

Rosemary Chicken

- Brush a 5-ounce boneless, skinless chicken breast with 1 teaspoon each of olive oil, lemon juice and rosemary. Grill or bake.

Fresh produce	Whole grains	Meat & dairy

Frozen goods	Canned goods	Miscellaneous

WEEK 2 PLANNER

SHOPPING LIST

QUICK TIP:

Create your shopping list for the week before going to the grocery store. You'll have all the ingredients on hand at the time you prepare a meal.

Fresh produce	Whole grains
asparagus	medium whole-wheat pasta shells
cherry tomatoes	
1 green pepper	brown rice
1 bunch green onions	1 loaf rye bre
green beans	bag of pitas
blueberries	
3 oranges	
4 apples	

▲

Add to your Shopping List as you plan your menus for the week.

TODAY'S DATE:

TODAY'S GOAL:

NOTES ABOUT TODAY:

WHAT I ATE TODAY:

Number of servings per food group

Time	Food item	Amount	V	F	C	PD	Ft	S

GLUCOSE READINGS:

A.M. fasting	P.M. before dinner

TODAY'S ACTIVITIES:

	🕐 Time
Total time (in minutes)	

WEEK 2

DAY 1

MOTIVATION TIP:

Increase your chances of sticking to your walking program by getting a walking buddy. A companion can help keep you motivated and make you feel safer.

KEY:

V	Vegetables
F	Fruits
C	Carbohydrates
PD	Protein/Dairy
Ft	Fats
S	Sweets

Sweets — 75 calories a day or 525 calories a week

← Write in your calories here.

Fats

Protein/Dairy

Carbohydrates

Fruits

Vegetables

WHAT I ATE TODAY FROM THE PYRAMID:

Check off the circles in the food group servings above as you record food and beverage items in the table at left. For sweets, give your best estimate of the total number of calories for the day.

TODAY'S DATE:

TODAY'S GOAL:

NOTES ABOUT TODAY:

WHAT I ATE TODAY:

Number of servings per food group

🕐 Time	Food item	Amount	V	F	C	PD	Ft	S

GLUCOSE READINGS:

A.M. fasting	P.M. before dinner

TODAY'S ACTIVITIES:

🕐 Time

Total time (in minutes)	

MOTIVATION TIP:

When you feel lonely, do you turn to food for comfort? When you're with friends, do you tend to overeat? Make a list of unhealthy behaviors and think of ways to change those behaviors.

KEY:

- **V** Vegetables
- **F** Fruits
- **C** Carbohydrates
- **PD** Protein/Dairy
- **Ft** Fats
- **S** Sweets

Sweets — 75 calories a day or 525 calories a week
→ Write in your calories here.

Fats

Protein/Dairy

Carbohydrates

Fruits

Vegetables

WHAT I ATE TODAY FROM THE PYRAMID:

Check off the circles in the food group servings above as you record food and beverage items in the table at left. For sweets, give your best estimate of the total number of calories for the day.

TODAY'S DATE:

TODAY'S GOAL:

NOTES ABOUT TODAY:

WHAT I ATE TODAY: Number of servings per food group

⏺ Time	Food item	Amount	V	F	C	PD	Ft	S

GLUCOSE READINGS:

A.M. fasting	P.M. before dinner

TODAY'S ACTIVITIES:

Time

Total time (in minutes)	

MOTIVATION TIP:
Keep foods that you crave out of the house or, at least, out of your sight. If you feel you must have a package of chocolate chips in the house, tuck them away in the back of a cupboard.

KEY:
- **V** Vegetables
- **F** Fruits
- **C** Carbohydrates
- **PD** Protein/Dairy
- **Ft** Fats
- **S** Sweets

Sweets — 75 calories a day or 525 calories a week
← Write in your calories here.

Fats

Protein/Dairy

Carbohydrates

Fruits

Vegetables

WHAT I ATE TODAY FROM THE PYRAMID:

Check off the circles in the food group servings above as you record food and beverage items in the table at left. For sweets, give your best estimate of the total number of calories for the day.

TODAY'S DATE:

TODAY'S GOAL:

NOTES ABOUT TODAY:

WHAT I ATE TODAY: **Number of servings per food group**

🕐 Time	Food item	Amount	V	F	C	PD	Ft	S

GLUCOSE READINGS:

A.M. fasting	P.M. before dinner

TODAY'S ACTIVITIES:

	🕐 Time
Total time (in minutes)	

MOTIVATION TIP:
Try out a new activity that you've always wanted to do. Base your decision on personal appeal and not necessarily on what you think will help you lose weight.

KEY:

V	Vegetables
F	Fruits
C	Carbohydrates
PD	Protein/Dairy
Ft	Fats
S	Sweets

Sweets — 75 calories a day or 525 calories a week
Write in your calories here.

Fats

Protein/Dairy

Carbohydrates

Fruits

Vegetables

WHAT I ATE TODAY FROM THE PYRAMID:
Check off the circles in the food group servings above as you record food and beverage items in the table at left. For sweets, give your best estimate of the total number of calories for the day.

TODAY'S DATE:

TODAY'S GOAL:

NOTES ABOUT TODAY:

WHAT I ATE TODAY: Number of servings per food group

⊕ Time	Food item	Amount	V	F	C	PD	Ft	S

GLUCOSE READINGS:

A.M. fasting	P.M. before dinner

TODAY'S ACTIVITIES: ⏱ **Time**

Total time (in minutes)	

MOTIVATION TIP:

Look for ways to make a favorite recipe more nutritious. This might include reducing the amount of sugar you add, using fat-free products and substituting legumes for meat.

KEY:

- **V** Vegetables
- **F** Fruits
- **C** Carbohydrates
- **PD** Protein/Dairy
- **Ft** Fats
- **S** Sweets

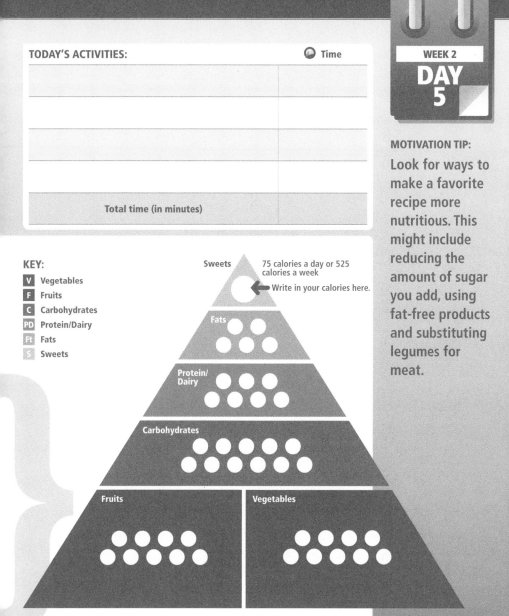

Sweets — 75 calories a day or 525 calories a week

Write in your calories here.

Fats

Protein/Dairy

Carbohydrates

Fruits

Vegetables

WHAT I ATE TODAY FROM THE PYRAMID:

Check off the circles in the food group servings above as you record food and beverage items in the table at left. For sweets, give your best estimate of the total number of calories for the day.

TODAY'S DATE:

TODAY'S GOAL:

NOTES ABOUT TODAY:

WHAT I ATE TODAY: Number of servings per food group

⏲ Time	Food item	Amount	V	F	C	PD	Ft	S

GLUCOSE READINGS:

A.M. fasting	P.M. before dinner

TODAY'S ACTIVITIES:

⏱ **Time**

Total time (in minutes)	

MOTIVATION TIP:
Keeping a positive attitude about exercise is important for success. If you start thinking, "Exercise is boring" or "Exercise takes too much time," you'll quickly lose motivation.

KEY:
- **V** Vegetables
- **F** Fruits
- **C** Carbohydrates
- **PD** Protein/Dairy
- **Ft** Fats
- **S** Sweets

Sweets
75 calories a day or 525 calories a week
← Write in your calories here.

Fats

Protein/Dairy

Carbohydrates

Fruits

Vegetables

WHAT I ATE TODAY FROM THE PYRAMID:
Check off the circles in the food group servings above as you record food and beverage items in the table at left. For sweets, give your best estimate of the total number of calories for the day.

TODAY'S DATE:

TODAY'S GOAL:

NOTES ABOUT TODAY:
It's weigh-in day ~ record my weight in the weekly Review and the Weight Record.

WHAT I ATE TODAY:

Number of servings per food group

Time	Food item	Amount	V	F	C	PD	Ft	S

GLUCOSE READINGS:

A.M. fasting	P.M. before dinner

TODAY'S ACTIVITIES:　　　　　　　　　⏱ Time

Total time (in minutes)	

REMINDER:

Record your weight for today in the weekly Review and the Weight Record.

KEY:

- **V** Vegetables
- **F** Fruits
- **C** Carbohydrates
- **PD** Protein/Dairy
- **Ft** Fats
- **S** Sweets

Sweets — 75 calories a day or 525 calories a week

◀ Write in your calories here.

Fats

Protein/Dairy

Carbohydrates

Fruits

Vegetables

WHAT I ATE TODAY FROM THE PYRAMID:

Check off the circles in the food group servings above as you record food and beverage items in the table at left. For sweets, give your best estimate of the total number of calories for the day.

My start weight	
Minus my weight today	
= Equals my weight change	

I FEEL:
- Terrific
- Good
- So-so
- Discouraged
- Like giving up

I'M MOST PROUD OF:

WHAT WORKED WELL:

WHAT DIDN'T WORK AS WELL:

DID I REACH MY SERVINGS GOALS FOR THIS WEEK?

Food group	Daily servings	Day 1	Day 2	Day 3	Day 4	Day 5	Day 6	Day 7
Vegetables		○	○	○	○	○	○	○
Fruits		○	○	○	○	○	○	○
Carbohydrates		○	○	○	○	○	○	○
Protein/Dairy		○	○	○	○	○	○	○
Fats		○	○	○	○	○	○	○
Sweets		○	○	○	○	○	○	○

DIRECTIONS:
1. Write your daily serving goals for each food group in the table above.
2. Compare the serving totals that you recorded for each day of the past week with your goals.
3. Check off the circles in the table above if your serving totals have met your goals.

CHANGES IN MY BLOOD SUGAR (GLUCOSE) READINGS:

NEW FOODS OR ACTIVITIES I WOULD LIKE TO TRY:

REMINDER: Calculate your weight change in this Review and record it in the Weight Record.

HOW MANY STEPS A DAY DID I TAKE (IF I USED A PEDOMETER)?

Day 1	Day 2	Day 3	Day 4	Day 5	Day 6	Day 7

HOW MANY MINUTES A DAY WAS I ACTIVE?

DIRECTIONS:
1. Add a dot for your total minutes of activity for each day of last week.
2. Connect each dot on the chart with a line.

See a sample chart to the right. →

The samples above show how you can fill out your servings goals table and your activity chart for your weekly Review.

Day	Breakfast	Lunch	Dinner	Snack
EXAMPLE	cereal banana	spaghetti fruit salad	tuna wrap baby carrots	crackers and cheese
1				
2				
3				
4				
5				
6				
7				

Exercise and activities	Events and special plans
swim class @ 11am walk to work	kids ballgame @ 6pm note: supper will be on the go

WEEK AT A GLANCE

USING THE PLANNER:

Organize your plans for meals, activities and exercise in the coming week. Note upcoming events that may affect your weight program, such as travel, eating out, social occasions and vacations.

MAIN MEAL OR MEALS OF THE DAY	HOW MUCH

EASY AS 1, 2, 3:

This page allows you to check how well a meal meets your recommended servings goals.

1. Write down what you're planning to eat for this meal (or for the entire day).

2. Calculate the number of servings based on how much you're planning to eat.

3. Be sure to include the food items from your menu in your Shopping List.

PYRAMID SERVINGS FOR THIS MEAL

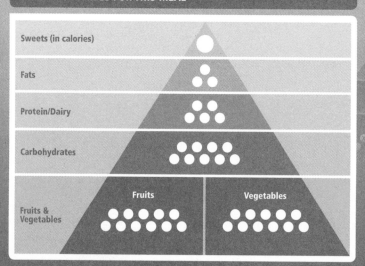

Sweets (in calories)

Fats

Protein/Dairy

Carbohydrates

Fruits & Vegetables — Fruits — Vegetables

◀ Check off the number of servings on the pyramid at left.

WEEK 3 PLANNER

MEAL PLANNER

MAIN MEAL OR MEALS OF THE DAY	HOW MUCH

EASY AS 1, 2, 3:

This page allows you to check how well a meal meets your recommended servings goals.

1. Write down what you're planning to eat for this meal (or for the entire day).

2. Calculate the number of servings based on how much you're planning to eat.

3. Be sure to include the food items from your menu in your Shopping List.

PYRAMID SERVINGS FOR THIS MEAL

◀ Check off the number of servings on the pyramid at left.

Live It!

MENU FOR THE DAY

BREAKFAST
1 whole-grain bagel
3 tbsp. fat-free cream cheese
1 medium orange
Calorie-free beverage

V	F	C	PD	Ft	S
0	1	2	0	1	0

DINNER
1 serving Beef Kebab
3 baby, red-skinned potatoes
1 large kiwi fruit
Calorie-free beverage

V	F	C	PD	Ft	S
2	1	1	2	0	0

LUNCH
Smoked Turkey Wrap
Cucumber and Tomato Salad
1 small apple
Calorie-free beverage

V	F	C	PD	Ft	S
2	1	1	1	1	0

SNACK
*1 serving favorite vegetable
2 tbsp. low-fat vegetable dip

V	F	C	PD	Ft	S
1	0	0	0	1	0

*The serving size stated is the minimum amount. Eat as much as you wish.

QUICK TIP:
The menu on this page demonstrates how you can plan your own daily menus. Feel free to include this sample on one of your days.

LUNCH RECIPE

Smoked Turkey Wrap

- Place 3 ounces of thin-sliced smoked turkey, shredded lettuce, sliced tomato and onion on a 6-inch tortilla. Top with 2 tablespoons of low-fat Western dressing. Roll up tortilla.

LUNCH RECIPE

Cucumber and Tomato Salad

- Combine 1 cup of thinly sliced cucumber and 8 cherry tomatoes, halved. Add balsamic, rice wine or herb-flavored vinegar to taste.

DINNER RECIPE

Beef Kebabs

- Place 3 ounces of marinated cubed round steak and a total of 2 cups diced fresh mushrooms, tomatoes, green peppers and onions on skewers. Broil or grill.

Fresh produce	Whole grains	Meat & dairy

Frozen goods	Canned goods	Miscellaneous

QUICK TIP:

Create your shopping list for the week before going to the grocery store. You'll have all the ingredients on hand at the time you prepare a meal.

Fresh produce	Whole grains
3 medium oranges	whole-grain bagels
4 apples	whole-wheat tortillas
kiwi fruit	1 loaf whole-wheat bread
red-skinned potatoes	8 oz package spaghetti
lettuce	
1 large tomato	
8 cherry tomatoes	
red onion	

▲

Add to your Shopping List as you plan your menus for the week.

TODAY'S DATE:

TODAY'S GOAL:

NOTES ABOUT TODAY:

WHAT I ATE TODAY: Number of servings per food group

⏱ Time	Food item	Amount	V	F	C	PD	Ft	S

GLUCOSE READINGS:

A.M. fasting	P.M. before dinner

TODAY'S ACTIVITIES:

	⏱ Time
Total time (in minutes)	

MOTIVATION TIP:
For best control of your blood sugar, don't "make up" servings. If you miss your target one day, don't add or skip servings the next. Start each day new, aiming for your target number of servings each day.

KEY:

- **V** Vegetables
- **F** Fruits
- **C** Carbohydrates
- **PD** Protein/Dairy
- **Ft** Fats
- **S** Sweets

Sweets

75 calories a day or 525 calories a week

← Write in your calories here.

Fats

Protein/Dairy

Carbohydrates

Fruits

Vegetables

WHAT I ATE TODAY FROM THE PYRAMID:

Check off the circles in the food group servings above as you record food and beverage items in the table at left. For sweets, give your best estimate of the total number of calories for the day.

TODAY'S DATE:

TODAY'S GOAL:

NOTES ABOUT TODAY:

WHAT I ATE TODAY:

Number of servings per food group

⏱ Time	Food item	Amount	V	F	C	PD	Ft	S

GLUCOSE READINGS:

A.M. fasting	P.M. before dinner

TODAY'S ACTIVITIES:

	⏱ **Time**
Total time (in minutes)	

WEEK 3

DAY
2

MOTIVATION TIP:
Rather than dwell on what you can't eat, focus on what you can eat. Granted, you may no longer be able to eat a large bowl of ice cream every evening, but you can have ice cream on occasion.

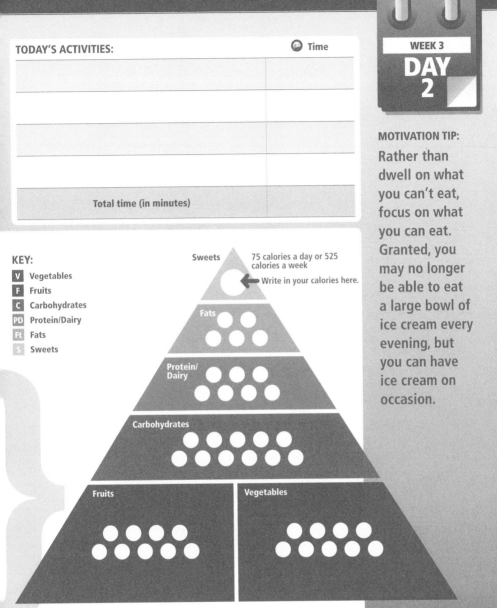

KEY:

V	Vegetables
F	Fruits
C	Carbohydrates
PD	Protein/Dairy
Ft	Fats
S	Sweets

Sweets — 75 calories a day or 525 calories a week
← Write in your calories here.

Fats

Protein/Dairy

Carbohydrates

Fruits

Vegetables

WHAT I ATE TODAY FROM THE PYRAMID:
Check off the circles in the food group servings above as you record food and beverage items in the table at left. For sweets, give your best estimate of the total number of calories for the day.

TODAY'S DATE:

TODAY'S GOAL:

NOTES ABOUT TODAY:

WHAT I ATE TODAY: **Number of servings per food group**

Time	Food item	Amount	V	F	C	PD	Ft	S

GLUCOSE READINGS:

A.M. fasting	P.M. before dinner

TODAY'S ACTIVITIES:

🕐 Time

Total time (in minutes)	

MOTIVATION TIP:

If your schedule is full, you can still find time to exercise for brief periods during the day. For example, do three 10-minute sessions in place of one 30-minute session.

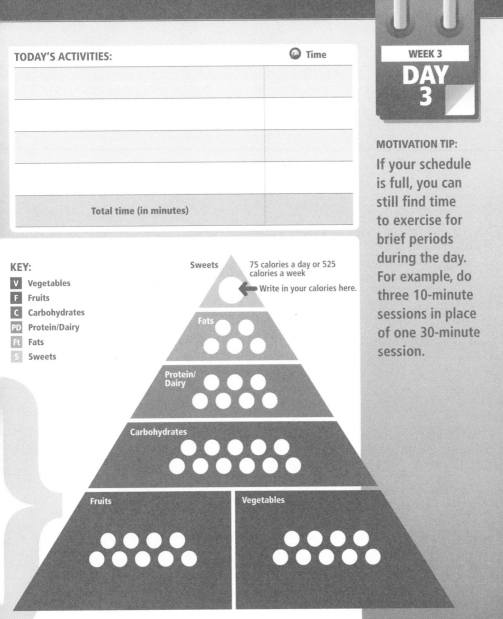

KEY:

- **V** Vegetables
- **F** Fruits
- **C** Carbohydrates
- **PD** Protein/Dairy
- **Ft** Fats
- **S** Sweets

Sweets

75 calories a day or 525 calories a week

← Write in your calories here.

Fats

Protein/ Dairy

Carbohydrates

Fruits

Vegetables

WHAT I ATE TODAY FROM THE PYRAMID:

Check off the circles in the food group servings above as you record food and beverage items in the table at left. For sweets, give your best estimate of the total number of calories for the day.

TODAY'S DATE:

TODAY'S GOAL:

NOTES ABOUT TODAY:

WHAT I ATE TODAY:

Number of servings per food group

Time	Food item	Amount	V	F	C	PD	Ft	S

GLUCOSE READINGS:

A.M. fasting	P.M. before dinner

TODAY'S ACTIVITIES: ⏱ Time

Total time (in minutes)	

MOTIVATION TIP:

Give yourself some slack. For example, it's OK to take a day off from exercising now and then — if you feel you really need it. You're not in exercise boot camp.

KEY:
- V Vegetables
- F Fruits
- C Carbohydrates
- PD Protein/Dairy
- Ft Fats
- S Sweets

Sweets 75 calories a day or 525 calories a week
← Write in your calories here.

Fats

Protein/Dairy

Carbohydrates

Fruits   Vegetables

WHAT I ATE TODAY FROM THE PYRAMID:
Check off the circles in the food group servings above as you record food and beverage items in the table at left. For sweets, give your best estimate of the total number of calories for the day.

TODAY'S DATE:

TODAY'S GOAL:

NOTES ABOUT TODAY:

WHAT I ATE TODAY:

Number of servings per food group

⏱ Time	Food item	Amount	V	F	C	PD	Ft	S

GLUCOSE READINGS:

A.M. fasting	P.M. before dinner

TODAY'S ACTIVITIES:

🕐 **Time**

Total time (in minutes)	

KEY:
- V Vegetables
- F Fruits
- C Carbohydrates
- PD Protein/Dairy
- Ft Fats
- S Sweets

Sweets

75 calories a day or 525 calories a week

← Write in your calories here.

Fats

Protein/ Dairy

Carbohydrates

Fruits

Vegetables

WHAT I ATE TODAY FROM THE PYRAMID:

Check off the circles in the food group servings above as you record food and beverage items in the table at left. For sweets, give your best estimate of the total number of calories for the day.

TODAY'S DATE:

TODAY'S GOAL:

NOTES ABOUT TODAY:

WHAT I ATE TODAY: **Number of servings per food group**

⏱ Time	Food item	Amount	V	F	C	PD	Ft	S

GLUCOSE READINGS:

A.M. fasting	P.M. before dinner

TODAY'S ACTIVITIES:

🕐 **Time**

Total time (in minutes)	

KEY:

- V Vegetables
- F Fruits
- C Carbohydrates
- PD Protein/Dairy
- Ft Fats
- S Sweets

Sweets — 75 calories a day or 525 calories a week

← Write in your calories here.

Fats

Protein/Dairy

Carbohydrates

Fruits

Vegetables

WHAT I ATE TODAY FROM THE PYRAMID:

Check off the circles in the food group servings above as you record food and beverage items in the table at left. For sweets, give your best estimate of the total number of calories for the day.

TODAY'S DATE:

TODAY'S GOAL:

NOTES ABOUT TODAY:
It's weigh-in day ~ record my weight in the weekly Review and the Weight Record.

WHAT I ATE TODAY:

Number of servings per food group

⏱ Time	Food item	Amount	V	F	C	PD	Ft	S

GLUCOSE READINGS:

A.M. fasting	P.M. before dinner

TODAY'S ACTIVITIES:

🕐 **Time**

Total time (in minutes)	

REMINDER:

Record your weight for today in the weekly Review and the Weight Record.

KEY:

- **V** Vegetables
- **F** Fruits
- **C** Carbohydrates
- **PD** Protein/Dairy
- **Ft** Fats
- **S** Sweets

Sweets — 75 calories a day or 525 calories a week

Write in your calories here.

Fats

Protein/ Dairy

Carbohydrates

Fruits

Vegetables

WHAT I ATE TODAY FROM THE PYRAMID:

Check off the circles in the food group servings above as you record food and beverage items in the table at left. For sweets, give your best estimate of the total number of calories for the day.

My start weight _____

Minus my weight today _____

= Equals my weight change _____

I FEEL:
- Terrific
- Good
- So-so
- Discouraged
- Like giving up

I'M MOST PROUD OF:

WHAT WORKED WELL:

WHAT DIDN'T WORK AS WELL:

DID I REACH MY SERVINGS GOALS FOR THIS WEEK?

Food group	Daily servings	Day 1	Day 2	Day 3	Day 4	Day 5	Day 6	Day 7
Vegetables		○	○	○	○	○	○	○
Fruits		○	○	○	○	○	○	○
Carbohydrates		○	○	○	○	○	○	○
Protein/Dairy		○	○	○	○	○	○	○
Fats		○	○	○	○	○	○	○
Sweets		○	○	○	○	○	○	○

DIRECTIONS:
1. Write your daily serving goals for each food group in the table above.
2. Compare the serving totals that you recorded for each day of the past week with your goals.
3. Check off the circles in the table above if your serving totals have met your goals.

CHANGES IN MY BLOOD SUGAR (GLUCOSE) READINGS:

NEW FOODS OR ACTIVITIES I WOULD LIKE TO TRY:

REMINDER:
Calculate your weight change in this Review and record it in the Weight Record.

HOW MANY STEPS A DAY DID I TAKE (IF I USED A PEDOMETER)?

Day 1	Day 2	Day 3	Day 4	Day 5	Day 6	Day 7

DID I REACH MY SERVINGS GOALS FOR THIS

Food group	Daily servings	Day 1	D
Vegetables	4+	✔	
Fruits	3+		
Carbohydrates	4	✔	
Protein/Dairy	3	✔	
Fats	3		✔

HOW MANY MINUTES A DAY WAS I ACTIVE?

DIRECTIONS:
1. Add a dot for your total minutes of activity for each day of last week.
2. Connect each dot on the chart with a line.

See a sample chart to the right. →

The samples above show how you can fill out your servings goals table and your activity chart for your weekly Review.

Day	Breakfast	Lunch	Dinner	Snack
EXAMPLE	cereal banana	spaghetti fruit salad	tuna wrap baby carrots	crackers and cheese
1				
2				
3				
4				
5				
6				
7				

Exercise and activities	Events and special plans
swim class @ 11am walk to work	kids ballgame @ 6pm note: supper will be on the go

WEEK AT A GLANCE

USING THE PLANNER:

Organize your plans for meals, activities and exercise in the coming week. Note upcoming events that may affect your weight program, such as travel, eating out, social occasions and vacations.

WEEK 4 PLANNER

MEAL PLANNER

MAIN MEAL OR MEALS OF THE DAY	HOW MUCH

EASY AS 1, 2, 3:

This page allows you to check how well a meal meets your recommended servings goals.

1. Write down what you're planning to eat for this meal (or for the entire day).

2. Calculate the number of servings based on how much you're planning to eat.

3. Be sure to include the food items from your menu in your Shopping List.

PYRAMID SERVINGS FOR THIS MEAL

Sweets (in calories)

Fats

Protein/Dairy

Carbohydrates

Fruits

Vegetables

Fruits & Vegetables

75

◀ Check off the number of servings on the pyramid at left.

MAIN MEAL OR MEALS OF THE DAY	HOW MUCH

EASY AS 1, 2, 3:

This page allows you to check how well a meal meets your recommended servings goals.

1. Write down what you're planning to eat for this meal (or for the entire day).

2. Calculate the number of servings based on how much you're planning to eat.

3. Be sure to include the food items from your menu in your Shopping List.

PYRAMID SERVINGS FOR THIS MEAL

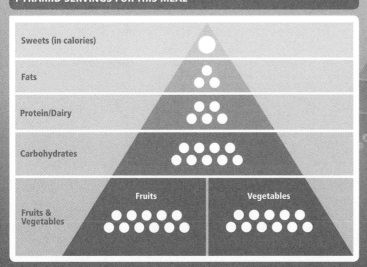

Sweets (in calories)

Fats

Protein/Dairy

Carbohydrates

Fruits & Vegetables — Fruits — Vegetables

‹ Check off the number of servings on the pyramid at left.

MENU &
RECIPE

MENU FOR THE DAY

BREAKFAST
½ c. cooked oatmeal
2 tbsp. raisins
1 c. skim milk
Calorie-free beverage

V	F	C	PD	Ft	S
0	1	1	1	0	0

DINNER
¼ Classic Tomato-Basil Pizza
*½ c. baby carrots
*¼ small cantaloupe
Calorie-free beverage

V	F	C	PD	Ft	S
2	1	2	2	0	0

LUNCH
Southwestern Salad
½ whole-grain pita bread
Calorie-free beverage

V	F	C	PD	Ft	S
2	1	1	1	2	0

SNACK
7 whole almonds

V	F	C	PD	Ft	S
0	0	0	0	1	0

*The serving size stated is the minimum amount. Eat as much as you wish.

QUICK TIP:

The menu on this page demonstrates how you can plan your own daily menus. Feel free to include this sample on one of your days.

LUNCH RECIPE

Southwestern Salad

- Top 2 cups shredded lettuce with 2½ ounces shredded cooked chicken, 1 cup chopped green peppers and onions, ½ cup crushed pineapple, ⅙ avocado and 2 tablespoons of reduced-calorie Western dressing.

DINNER RECIPE

Classic Tomato-Basil Pizza

- Top a prepared 14-inch pizza crust with 1 cup diced plum tomatoes, fresh basil and 1⅓ cup low-fat shredded mozzarella cheese. Bake at 400 F about 10 minutes.

WEEK 4 PLANNER

SHOPPING LIST

Fresh produce	Whole grains	Meat & dairy

Frozen goods	Canned goods	Miscellaneous

QUICK TIP:

Create your shopping list for the week before going to the grocery store. You'll have all the ingredients on hand at the time you prepare a meal.

Fresh produce	Whole grai
1 bag baby carrots	old-fashioned oatmeal
lettuce	bag of whole-grain pitas
2 green peppers	
1 red onion	1 package English muf
avocado	
pineapple	whole-grain cereal
cantaloupe	

▲
Add to your Shopping List as you plan your menus for the week.

TODAY'S DATE:

TODAY'S GOAL:

NOTES ABOUT TODAY:

WHAT I ATE TODAY: Number of servings per food group

⏰ Time	Food item	Amount	V	F	C	PD	Ft	S

GLUCOSE READINGS:

A.M. fasting	P.M. before dinner

TODAY'S ACTIVITIES:

⏱ **Time**

Total time (in minutes)	

MOTIVATION TIP:

Try not to focus only on physical exertion while you exercise. Think of pleasant thoughts or enjoyable things to do at the same time that you're physically active.

KEY:

V	Vegetables
F	Fruits
C	Carbohydrates
PD	Protein/Dairy
Ft	Fats
S	Sweets

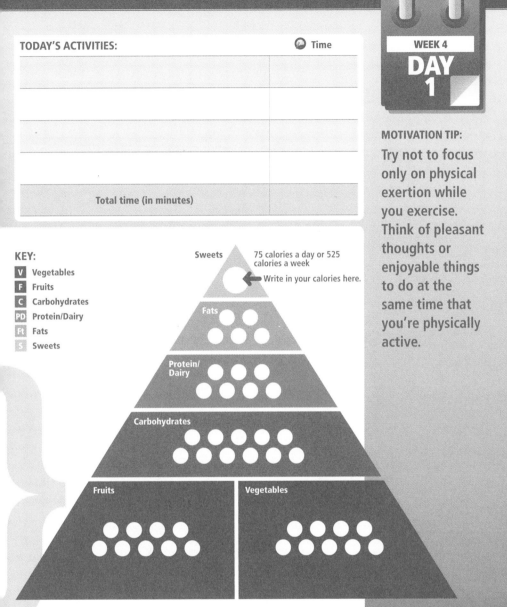

Sweets — 75 calories a day or 525 calories a week
← Write in your calories here.

Fats

Protein/Dairy

Carbohydrates

Fruits

Vegetables

WHAT I ATE TODAY FROM THE PYRAMID:

Check off the circles in the food group servings above as you record food and beverage items in the table at left. For sweets, give your best estimate of the total number of calories for the day.

TODAY'S DATE:

TODAY'S GOAL:

NOTES ABOUT TODAY:

WHAT I ATE TODAY: Number of servings per food group

⏱ Time	Food item	Amount	V	F	C	PD	Ft	S

GLUCOSE READINGS:

A.M. fasting	P.M. before dinner

TODAY'S ACTIVITIES:

	Time
Total time (in minutes)	

WEEK 4

DAY 2

MOTIVATION TIP:
The urge to eat can often be due to a certain mood and not to physical hunger. When the mood sets in, try to distract yourself by going for a walk, calling a friend or running an errand.

KEY:

- **V** Vegetables
- **F** Fruits
- **C** Carbohydrates
- **PD** Protein/Dairy
- **Ft** Fats
- **S** Sweets

Sweets

75 calories a day or 525 calories a week

← Write in your calories here.

Fats

Protein/Dairy

Carbohydrates

Fruits

Vegetables

WHAT I ATE TODAY FROM THE PYRAMID:
Check off the circles in the food group servings above as you record food and beverage items in the table at left. For sweets, give your best estimate of the total number of calories for the day.

TODAY'S DATE:

TODAY'S GOAL:

NOTES ABOUT TODAY:

WHAT I ATE TODAY: Number of servings per food group

⏱ Time	Food item	Amount	V	F	C	PD	Ft	S

GLUCOSE READINGS:

A.M. fasting	P.M. before dinner

TODAY'S ACTIVITIES:

	⏱ Time
Total time (in minutes)	

MOTIVATION TIP:

Accept the fact that on some days, you'll have setbacks. Rather than give up on your program entirely, simply start fresh on the next day. Believe in yourself.

KEY:

- **V** Vegetables
- **F** Fruits
- **C** Carbohydrates
- **PD** Protein/Dairy
- **Ft** Fats
- **S** Sweets

Sweets — 75 calories a day or 525 calories a week

Write in your calories here.

Fats

Protein/Dairy

Carbohydrates

Fruits

Vegetables

WHAT I ATE TODAY FROM THE PYRAMID:
Check off the circles in the food group servings above as you record food and beverage items in the table at left. For sweets, give your best estimate of the total number of calories for the day.

TODAY'S DATE:

TODAY'S GOAL:

NOTES ABOUT TODAY:

WHAT I ATE TODAY: Number of servings per food group

⏱ Time	Food item	Amount	V	F	C	PD	Ft	S

GLUCOSE READINGS:

A.M. fasting	P.M. before dinner

TODAY'S ACTIVITIES:

⏱ Time

Total time (in minutes)	

MOTIVATION TIP:
You don't have to like all vegetables and fruits, just some of them. To increase the number of servings you eat, try preparing them in different ways, for example, grilling vegetables or topping your cereal with fruit.

KEY:

V Vegetables
F Fruits
C Carbohydrates
PD Protein/Dairy
Ft Fats
S Sweets

Sweets

75 calories a day or 525 calories a week

Write in your calories here.

Fats

Protein/Dairy

Carbohydrates

Fruits

Vegetables

WHAT I ATE TODAY FROM THE PYRAMID:
Check off the circles in the food group servings above as you record food and beverage items in the table at left. For sweets, give your best estimate of the total number of calories for the day.

TODAY'S DATE:

TODAY'S GOAL:

NOTES ABOUT TODAY:

WHAT I ATE TODAY: Number of servings per food group

⏱ Time	Food item	Amount	V	F	C	PD	Ft	S

GLUCOSE READINGS:

A.M. fasting	P.M. before dinner

TODAY'S ACTIVITIES:

⏱ **Time**

Total time (in minutes)	

MOTIVATION TIP:

Don't let unsupportive friends distract you from your goals. Try to be around people who share similar goals and who are willing to provide support.

KEY:

V Vegetables
F Fruits
C Carbohydrates
PD Protein/Dairy
Ft Fats
S Sweets

Sweets — 75 calories a day or 525 calories a week
← Write in your calories here.

Fats

Protein/Dairy

Carbohydrates

Fruits

Vegetables

WHAT I ATE TODAY FROM THE PYRAMID:
Check off the circles in the food group servings above as you record food and beverage items in the table at left. For sweets, give your best estimate of the total number of calories for the day.

TODAY'S DATE:

TODAY'S GOAL:

NOTES ABOUT TODAY:

WHAT I ATE TODAY:

Number of servings per food group

Time	Food item	Amount	V	F	C	PD	Ft	S

GLUCOSE READINGS:

A.M. fasting	P.M. before dinner

TODAY'S ACTIVITIES:

⏱ **Time**

Total time (in minutes)	

MOTIVATION TIP:
Try to eat three meals during the day, including a good breakfast. This can help prevent late-night snacking, simply because you won't be so hungry.

KEY:

V   Vegetables
F   Fruits
C   Carbohydrates
PD   Protein/Dairy
Ft   Fats
S   Sweets

Sweets — 75 calories a day or 525 calories a week
← Write in your calories here.

Fats

Protein/Dairy

Carbohydrates

Fruits

Vegetables

WHAT I ATE TODAY FROM THE PYRAMID:
Check off the circles in the food group servings above as you record food and beverage items in the table at left. For sweets, give your best estimate of the total number of calories for the day.

TODAY'S DATE:

TODAY'S GOAL:

NOTES ABOUT TODAY:
It's weigh-in day ~ record my weight in the weekly Review and the Weight Record.

WHAT I ATE TODAY:

Number of servings per food group

Time	Food item	Amount	V	F	C	PD	Ft	S

GLUCOSE READINGS:

A.M. fasting	P.M. before dinner

TODAY'S ACTIVITIES:

🕐 Time

Total time (in minutes)	

REMINDER: 🔍
Record your weight for today in the weekly Review and the Weight Record.

KEY:

- **V** Vegetables
- **F** Fruits
- **C** Carbohydrates
- **PD** Protein/Dairy
- **Ft** Fats
- **S** Sweets

Sweets

75 calories a day or 525 calories a week

◄ Write in your calories here.

Fats

Protein/Dairy

Carbohydrates

Fruits

Vegetables

WHAT I ATE TODAY FROM THE PYRAMID:

Check off the circles in the food group servings above as you record food and beverage items in the table at left. For sweets, give your best estimate of the total number of calories for the day.

Live It!

WEEK 4 · REVIEW Re-examine how your week went.

My start weight

Minus my weight today

= Equals my weight change

I FEEL:
- Terrific
- Good
- So-so
- Discouraged
- Like giving up

I'M MOST PROUD OF:

WHAT WORKED WELL:

WHAT DIDN'T WORK AS WELL:

DID I REACH MY SERVINGS GOALS FOR THIS WEEK?

Food group	Daily servings	Day 1	Day 2	Day 3	Day 4	Day 5	Day 6	Day 7
Vegetables		○	○	○	○	○	○	○
Fruits		○	○	○	○	○	○	○
Carbohydrates		○	○	○	○	○	○	○
Protein/Dairy		○	○	○	○	○	○	○
Fats		○	○	○	○	○	○	○
Sweets		○	○	○	○	○	○	○

DIRECTIONS:
1. Write your daily serving goals for each food group in the table above.
2. Compare the serving totals that you recorded for each day of the past week with your goals.
3. Check off the circles in the table above if your serving totals have met your goals.

CHANGES IN MY BLOOD SUGAR (GLUCOSE) READINGS:

NEW FOODS OR ACTIVITIES I WOULD LIKE TO TRY:

REMINDER: Calculate your weight change in this Review and record it in the Weight Record.

HOW MANY STEPS A DAY DID I TAKE (IF I USED A PEDOMETER)?

Day 1	Day 2	Day 3	Day 4	Day 5	Day 6	Day 7

HOW MANY MINUTES A DAY WAS I ACTIVE?

DIRECTIONS:

1. Add a dot for your total minutes of activity for each day of last week.
2. Connect each dot on the chart with a line.

See a sample chart to the right. →

The samples above show how you can fill out your servings goals table and your activity chart for your weekly Review.

Review **127**

Day	Breakfast	Lunch	Dinner	Snack
EXAMPLE	cereal banana	spaghetti fruit salad	tuna wrap baby carrots	crackers and cheese
1				
2				
3				
4				
5				
6				
7				

Exercise and activities	Events and special plans
swim class @ 11am walk to work	kids ballgame @ 6pm note: supper will be on the go

USING THE PLANNER:

Organize your plans for meals, activities and exercise in the coming week. Note upcoming events that may affect your weight program, such as travel, eating out, social occasions and vacations.

MAIN MEAL OR MEALS OF THE DAY	HOW MUCH

EASY AS 1, 2, 3:

This page allows you to check how well a meal meets your recommended servings goals.

1. Write down what you're planning to eat for this meal (or for the entire day).

2. Calculate the number of servings based on how much you're planning to eat.

3. Be sure to include the food items from your menu in your Shopping List.

PYRAMID SERVINGS FOR THIS MEAL

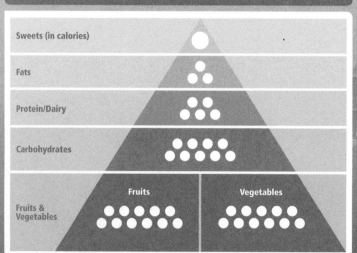

Sweets (in calories)	○
Fats	○○○
Protein/Dairy	○○○○
Carbohydrates	○○○○○ ○○○○
Fruits & Vegetables	**Fruits** ○○○○○ ○○○○○ **Vegetables** ○○○○○ ○○○○○

◄ Check off the number of servings on the pyramid at left.

MAIN MEAL OR MEALS OF THE DAY	HOW MUCH

EASY AS 1, 2, 3:

This page allows you to check how well a meal meets your recommended servings goals.

1. Write down what you're planning to eat for this meal (or for the entire day).

2. Calculate the number of servings based on how much you're planning to eat.

3. Be sure to include the food items from your menu in your Shopping List.

PYRAMID SERVINGS FOR THIS MEAL

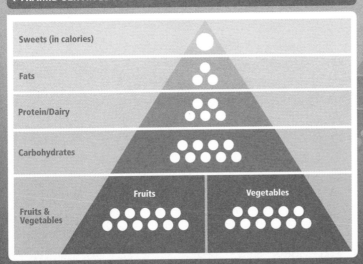

Sweets (in calories)	⚪
Fats	⚪⚪⚪
Protein/Dairy	⚪⚪⚪⚪⚪
Carbohydrates	⚪⚪⚪⚪⚪⚪⚪⚪
Fruits & Vegetables	**Fruits** ⚪⚪⚪⚪⚪⚪⚪⚪⚪⚪ **Vegetables** ⚪⚪⚪⚪⚪⚪⚪⚪⚪

75

◀ Check off the number of servings on the pyramid at left.

MENU FOR THE DAY

BREAKFAST

Omelet
1 slice whole-grain toast
1 tsp. trans fat-free margarine
1 small banana
Calorie-free beverage

V	F	C	PD	Ft	S
1	1	1	1	1	0

LUNCH

Bagel Sandwich
*2 c. raw vegetables
Calorie-free beverage

V	F	C	PD	Ft	S
2	0	2	1	1	0

DINNER

1 serving Chinese Noodles and
   Vegetables
½ c. pineapple chunks
1 c. skim milk
Calorie-free beverage

V	F	C	PD	Ft	S
2	1	1	1	1	0

SNACK

1 serving favorite fruit

V	F	C	PD	Ft	S
0	1	0	0	0	0

*The serving size stated is the minimum amount. Eat as much as you wish.

QUICK TIP:

The menu on this page demonstrates how you can plan your own daily menus. Feel free to include this sample on one of your days.

BREAKFAST RECIPE

Omelet

■ Mix ½ cup egg substitute with ½ cup diced onions, tomatoes, green peppers and mushrooms, and cook until set.

LUNCH RECIPE

Bagel Sandwich

■ Spread 1 whole-grain bagel with 1 tablespoon reduced-calorie mayonnaise. Top with 2 ounces lean ham, lettuce, tomato and onion slice.

DINNER RECIPE

Chinese Noodles and Vegetables

■ Prepare 1 package ramen noodles as directed. Rinse and set aside. Sauté 1 tablespoon grated ginger and 1 tablespoon chopped garlic in 1 tablespoon sesame oil and 1 tablespoon peanut oil. Add ½ cup broccoli florets and sauté 3 minutes. Add ½ cup of each: bean sprouts, fresh spinach and cherry tomato halves. Add noodles and toss. Sprinkle with chopped green onions and soy sauce.

Fresh produce	Whole grains	Meat & dairy

Frozen goods	Canned goods	Miscellaneous

WEEK 5 PLANNER

SHOPPING LIST

QUICK TIP:

Create your shopping list for the week before going to the grocery store. You'll have all the ingredients on hand at the time you prepare a meal.

Fresh produce	Whole grains
bananas	whole-grain bre
pineapple	whole-grain bagels
broccoli	whole-grain cereal
bean sprouts	
spinach	whole-wheat pasta shells
cherry tomatoes	
1 bunch green onions	

▲
Add to your Shopping List as you plan your menus for the week.

TODAY'S DATE:

TODAY'S GOAL:

NOTES ABOUT TODAY:

WHAT I ATE TODAY:

Number of servings per food group

Time	Food item	Amount	V	F	C	PD	Ft	S

GLUCOSE READINGS:

A.M. fasting	P.M. before dinner

TODAY'S ACTIVITIES:

	⏱ Time
Total time (in minutes)	

MOTIVATION TIP:
Make sure you're not skipping breakfast. If necessary, keep food handy that you can carry with you in the morning. Eat on the train or bus, or at work.

KEY:

V Vegetables
F Fruits
C Carbohydrates
PD Protein/Dairy
Ft Fats
S Sweets

Sweets
75 calories a day or 525 calories a week
Write in your calories here.

Fats

Protein/Dairy

Carbohydrates

Fruits

Vegetables

WHAT I ATE TODAY FROM THE PYRAMID:
Check off the circles in the food group servings above as you record food and beverage items in the table at left. For sweets, give your best estimate of the total number of calories for the day.

TODAY'S DATE:

TODAY'S GOAL:

NOTES ABOUT TODAY:

WHAT I ATE TODAY:

Number of servings per food group

Time	Food item	Amount	V	F	C	PD	Ft	S

GLUCOSE READINGS:

A.M. fasting	P.M. before dinner

TODAY'S ACTIVITIES:

🕐 **Time**

Total time (in minutes)	

MOTIVATION TIP:
Every bit of food you eat doesn't have to be an excellent source of nutrition. Your main goal is to choose foods that promote good health more often than you choose those that don't.

KEY:

V	Vegetables
F	Fruits
C	Carbohydrates
PD	Protein/Dairy
Ft	Fats
S	Sweets

Sweets

75 calories a day or 525 calories a week

← Write in your calories here.

Fats

Protein/ Dairy

Carbohydrates

Fruits   Vegetables

WHAT I ATE TODAY FROM THE PYRAMID:
Check off the circles in the food group servings above as you record food and beverage items in the table at left. For sweets, give your best estimate of the total number of calories for the day.

TODAY'S DATE:

TODAY'S GOAL:

NOTES ABOUT TODAY:

WHAT I ATE TODAY: Number of servings per food group

⏱ Time	Food item	Amount	V	F	C	PD	Ft	S

GLUCOSE READINGS:

A.M. fasting	P.M. before dinner

TODAY'S ACTIVITIES:

⏱ **Time**

Total time (in minutes)	

MOTIVATION TIP:
Make exercise a priority today. If you treat it as secondary, exercise will quickly drop to the bottom of your to-do list.

KEY:

V Vegetables
F Fruits
C Carbohydrates
PD Protein/Dairy
Ft Fats
S Sweets

Sweets   75 calories a day or 525 calories a week
← Write in your calories here.

Fats

Protein/Dairy

Carbohydrates

Fruits   Vegetables

WHAT I ATE TODAY FROM THE PYRAMID:
Check off the circles in the food group servings above as you record food and beverage items in the table at left. For sweets, give your best estimate of the total number of calories for the day.

TODAY'S DATE:

TODAY'S GOAL:

NOTES ABOUT TODAY:

WHAT I ATE TODAY: Number of servings per food group

🕐 Time	Food item	Amount	V	F	C	PD	Ft	S

GLUCOSE READINGS:

A.M. fasting	P.M. before dinner

TODAY'S ACTIVITIES:

⏱ **Time**

Total time (in minutes)	

MOTIVATION TIP:
Exercise should not be painful. Muscle soreness after exercise is common, but pain during exercise can be a signal of impending injury. Stop what you're doing and consult your doctor.

KEY:

- V Vegetables
- F Fruits
- C Carbohydrates
- PD Protein/Dairy
- Ft Fats
- S Sweets

Sweets

75 calories a day or 525 calories a week

← Write in your calories here.

Fats

Protein/Dairy

Carbohydrates

Fruits

Vegetables

WHAT I ATE TODAY FROM THE PYRAMID:
Check off the circles in the food group servings above as you record food and beverage items in the table at left. For sweets, give your best estimate of the total number of calories for the day.

TODAY'S DATE:

TODAY'S GOAL:

NOTES ABOUT TODAY:

WHAT I ATE TODAY: Number of servings per food group

⏱ Time	Food item	Amount	V	F	C	PD	Ft	S

GLUCOSE READINGS:

A.M. fasting	P.M. before dinner

TODAY'S ACTIVITIES:

⏱ Time

Total time (in minutes)	

MOTIVATION TIP:
Eating to ease stress almost always ends in overeating. Look for other ways to cope with stress, including exercise, regular mealtimes and getting enough sleep.

KEY:

- **V** Vegetables
- **F** Fruits
- **C** Carbohydrates
- **PD** Protein/Dairy
- **Ft** Fats
- **S** Sweets

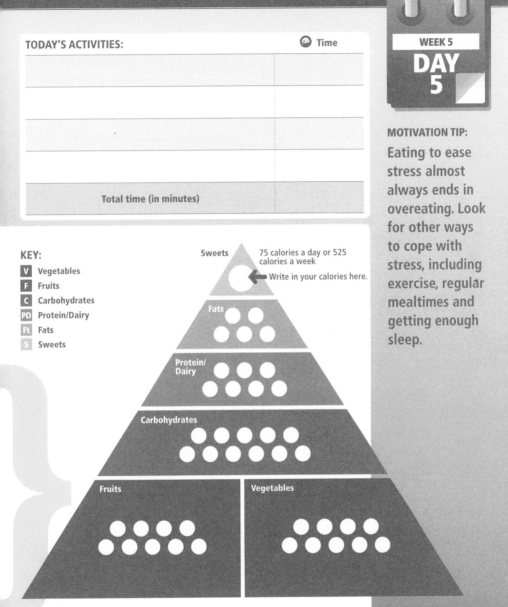

Sweets — 75 calories a day or 525 calories a week

Write in your calories here.

Fats

Protein/Dairy

Carbohydrates

Fruits

Vegetables

WHAT I ATE TODAY FROM THE PYRAMID:

Check off the circles in the food group servings above as you record food and beverage items in the table at left. For sweets, give your best estimate of the total number of calories for the day.

TODAY'S DATE:

TODAY'S GOAL:

NOTES ABOUT TODAY:

WHAT I ATE TODAY: Number of servings per food group

⏱ Time	Food item	Amount	V	F	C	PD	Ft	S

GLUCOSE READINGS:

A.M. fasting	P.M. before dinner

TODAY'S ACTIVITIES:

Time

Total time (in minutes)	

MOTIVATION TIP:
Keep your response to an eating or exercise lapse simple. Focus on the things you know you can do and avoid drastic changes. You'll soon get back on track.

KEY:
- V Vegetables
- F Fruits
- C Carbohydrates
- PD Protein/Dairy
- Ft Fats
- S Sweets

Sweets — 75 calories a day or 525 calories a week

Write in your calories here.

Fats

Protein/Dairy

Carbohydrates

Fruits

Vegetables

WHAT I ATE TODAY FROM THE PYRAMID:
Check off the circles in the food group servings above as you record food and beverage items in the table at left. For sweets, give your best estimate of the total number of calories for the day.

TODAY'S DATE:

TODAY'S GOAL:

NOTES ABOUT TODAY:
It's weigh-in day ~ record my weight in the weekly Review and the Weight Record.

WHAT I ATE TODAY:　　　　　　　　　　　　　Number of servings per food group

Time	Food item	Amount	V	F	C	PD	Ft	S

GLUCOSE READINGS:

A.M. fasting	P.M. before dinner

TODAY'S ACTIVITIES:

	Time
Total time (in minutes)	

REMINDER:
Record your weight for today in the weekly Review and the Weight Record.

KEY:

- **V** Vegetables
- **F** Fruits
- **C** Carbohydrates
- **PD** Protein/Dairy
- **Ft** Fats
- **S** Sweets

Sweets

75 calories a day or 525 calories a week

Write in your calories here.

Fats

Protein/ Dairy

Carbohydrates

Fruits

Vegetables

WHAT I ATE TODAY FROM THE PYRAMID:

Check off the circles in the food group servings above as you record food and beverage items in the table at left. For sweets, give your best estimate of the total number of calories for the day.

My start weight	
Minus my weight today	
= Equals my weight change	

I FEEL:
- Terrific
- Good
- So-so
- Discouraged
- Like giving up

I'M MOST PROUD OF:

WHAT WORKED WELL:

WHAT DIDN'T WORK AS WELL:

DID I REACH MY SERVINGS GOALS FOR THIS WEEK?

Food group	Daily servings	Day 1	Day 2	Day 3	Day 4	Day 5	Day 6	Day 7
Vegetables		○	○	○	○	○	○	○
Fruits		○	○	○	○	○	○	○
Carbohydrates		○	○	○	○	○	○	○
Protein/Dairy		○	○	○	○	○	○	○
Fats		○	○	○	○	○	○	○
Sweets		○	○	○	○	○	○	○

DIRECTIONS:

1. Write your daily serving goals for each food group in the table above.
2. Compare the serving totals that you recorded for each day of the past week with your goals.
3. Check off the circles in the table above if your serving totals have met your goals.

CHANGES IN MY BLOOD SUGAR (GLUCOSE) READINGS:

NEW FOODS OR ACTIVITIES I WOULD LIKE TO TRY:

REMINDER: Calculate your weight change in this Review and record it in the Weight Record.

HOW MANY STEPS A DAY DID I TAKE (IF I USED A PEDOMETER)?

Day 1	Day 2	Day 3	Day 4	Day 5	Day 6	Day 7

DID I REACH MY SERVINGS GOALS FOR THIS

Food group	Daily servings	Day 1	Da
Vegetables	4+	✔	
Fruits	3+		
Carbohydrates	4	✔	✔
Protein/Dairy	3	✔	✔
Fats	3		✔

HOW MANY MINUTES A DAY WAS I ACTIVE?

DIRECTIONS:
1. Add a dot for your total minutes of activity for each day of last week.
2. Connect each dot on the chart with a line.

See a sample chart to the right. →

The samples above show how you can fill out your servings goals table and your activity chart for your weekly Review.

Day	Breakfast	Lunch	Dinner	Snack
EXAMPLE	cereal banana	spaghetti fruit salad	tuna wrap baby carrots	crackers and cheese
1				
2				
3				
4				
5				
6				
7				

Exercise and activities	Events and special plans
swim class @ 11am walk to work	kids ballgame @ 6pm note: supper will be on the go

WEEK AT A GLANCE

USING THE PLANNER:

Organize your plans for meals, activities and exercise in the coming week. Note upcoming events that may affect your weight program, such as travel, eating out, social occasions and vacations.

MAIN MEAL OR MEALS OF THE DAY	HOW MUCH

EASY AS 1, 2, 3:

This page allows you to check how well a meal meets your recommended servings goals.

1. Write down what you're planning to eat for this meal (or for the entire day).
2. Calculate the number of servings based on how much you're planning to eat.
3. Be sure to include the food items from your menu in your Shopping List.

PYRAMID SERVINGS FOR THIS MEAL

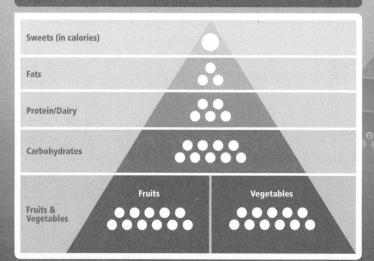

Sweets (in calories)

Fats

Protein/Dairy

Carbohydrates

Fruits

Vegetables

Fruits & Vegetables

◄ Check off the number of servings on the pyramid at left.

MAIN MEAL OR MEALS OF THE DAY	HOW MUCH

EASY AS 1, 2, 3:

This page allows you to check how well a meal meets your recommended servings goals.

1. Write down what you're planning to eat for this meal (or for the entire day).

2. Calculate the number of servings based on how much you're planning to eat.

3. Be sure to include the food items from your menu in your Shopping List.

PYRAMID SERVINGS FOR THIS MEAL

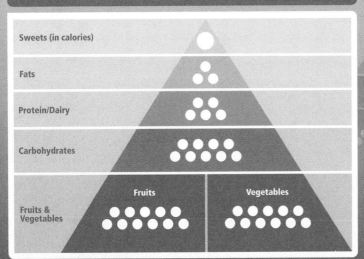

Sweets (in calories)	○
Fats	○○○
Protein/Dairy	○○○○○
Carbohydrates	○○○○○ ○○○○
Fruits & Vegetables	**Fruits** ○○○○○ ○○○○○ **Vegetables** ○○○○○ ○○○○○

◄ Check off the number of servings on the pyramid at left.

MENU FOR THE DAY

BREAKFAST
1 small muffin, any flavor
2 tsp. trans fat-free margarine
2 pear halves
Calorie-free beverage

V	F	C	PD	Ft	S
0	1	2	0	2	0

LUNCH
Chicken wrap
*1 medium tomato
1 medium apple
Calorie-free beverage

V	F	C	PD	Ft	S
1	1	1	1	1	0

DINNER
5 oz. lean pork, grilled or broiled
⅓ c. cooked brown rice
1 serving Sesame Asparagus and
    Carrot Stir-Fry
1 small slice angel food cake
1 c. berries
Calorie-free beverage

V	F	C	PD	Ft	S
2	1	1	2	1	1

SNACK
*1 serving favorite vegetable

V	F	C	PD	Ft	S
1	0	0	0	0	0

*The serving size stated is the minimum amount. Eat as much as you wish.

QUICK TIP:
The menu on this page demonstrates how you can plan your own daily menus. Feel free to include this sample on one of your days.

DINNER RECIPE

Sesame Asparagus and Carrot Stir-Fry (SERVES 6)

24 asparagus stalks
6   large carrots
¼   C. water
1   tbsp. grated fresh ginger
1   tbsp. reduced-sodium soy sauce
1½ tsp. sesame oil
1½ tbsp. sesame seeds, toasted

- Cut the asparagus into ½-inch-thick slices. Cut the carrots into ¼-inch-thick slices.

- Coat a wok or frying pan with cooking spray and place over high heat. Add the carrots and stir-fry for 4 minutes. Add the asparagus and water. Stir and toss to combine. Cover and cook until the vegetables are barely tender, about 2 minutes. Uncover and add the ginger. Stir-fry until remaining water evaporates, about 1 to 2 minutes.

- Add the soy sauce, sesame oil and sesame seeds. Stir-fry to coat the vegetables evenly. Dish onto individual plates and serve.

Fresh produce	Whole grains	Meat & dairy

Frozen goods	Canned goods	Miscellaneous

WEEK 6 PLANNER
SHOPPING LIST

QUICK TIP:

Create your shopping list for the week before going to the grocery store. You'll have all the ingredients on hand at the time you prepare a meal.

Fresh produce	Whole grains
1 medium tomato	brown rice
2 bunches asparagus	bran muffins
6 large carrots	1 loaf rye brea
pears	bag of pitas
raspberries	
3 medium apples	

Add to your Shopping List as you plan your menus for the week.

TODAY'S DATE:

TODAY'S GOAL:

NOTES ABOUT TODAY:

WHAT I ATE TODAY: Number of servings per food group

⏱ Time	Food item	Amount	V	F	C	PD	Ft	S

GLUCOSE READINGS:

A.M. fasting	P.M. before dinner

TODAY'S ACTIVITIES:

	⏱ Time
Total time (in minutes)	

MOTIVATION TIP:

Try listening to music while you exercise. Upbeat music can rev you up. It makes the workout seem easier and the time pass more quickly.

KEY:

V Vegetables
F Fruits
C Carbohydrates
PD Protein/Dairy
Ft Fats
S Sweets

Sweets — 75 calories a day or 525 calories a week
← Write in your calories here.

Fats

Protein/Dairy

Carbohydrates

Fruits   Vegetables

WHAT I ATE TODAY FROM THE PYRAMID:

Check off the circles in the food group servings above as you record food and beverage items in the table at left. For sweets, give your best estimate of the total number of calories for the day.

TODAY'S DATE:

TODAY'S GOAL:

NOTES ABOUT TODAY:

WHAT I ATE TODAY: Number of servings per food group

⏱ Time	Food item	Amount	V	F	C	PD	Ft	S

GLUCOSE READINGS:

A.M. fasting	P.M. before dinner

TODAY'S ACTIVITIES:

🕐 **Time**

Total time (in minutes)	

MOTIVATION TIP:
Don't shop on an empty stomach. Eat something before you go to the store. If you're hungry, it's harder to resist the bright packaging and enticing smells of many high-calorie foods.

KEY:

- **V** Vegetables
- **F** Fruits
- **C** Carbohydrates
- **PD** Protein/Dairy
- **Ft** Fats
- **S** Sweets

Sweets
75 calories a day or 525 calories a week
← Write in your calories here.

Fats

Protein/Dairy

Carbohydrates

Fruits

Vegetables

WHAT I ATE TODAY FROM THE PYRAMID:
Check off the circles in the food group servings above as you record food and beverage items in the table at left. For sweets, give your best estimate of the total number of calories for the day.

TODAY'S DATE:

TODAY'S GOAL:

NOTES ABOUT TODAY:

WHAT I ATE TODAY:

Number of servings per food group

Time	Food item	Amount	V	F	C	PD	Ft	S

GLUCOSE READINGS:

A.M. fasting	P.M. before dinner

TODAY'S ACTIVITIES: 🕐 Time

Total time (in minutes)	

MOTIVATION TIP:
Acknowledge
that you're
a person of
value who can
contribute to
your community
and to others,
regardless of
what you weigh.

KEY:

- **V** Vegetables
- **F** Fruits
- **C** Carbohydrates
- **PD** Protein/Dairy
- **Ft** Fats
- **S** Sweets

Sweets — 75 calories a day or 525 calories a week

← Write in your calories here.

Fats

Protein/Dairy

Carbohydrates

Fruits

Vegetables

WHAT I ATE TODAY FROM THE PYRAMID:
Check off the circles in the food group servings above as you record
food and beverage items in the table at left. For sweets, give your best
estimate of the total number of calories for the day.

TODAY'S DATE:

TODAY'S GOAL:

NOTES ABOUT TODAY:

WHAT I ATE TODAY:

Number of servings per food group

🕐 Time	Food item	Amount	V	F	C	PD	Ft	S

GLUCOSE READINGS:

A.M. fasting	P.M. before dinner

TODAY'S ACTIVITIES:

⏲ Time

Total time (in minutes)	

KEY:

V Vegetables
F Fruits
C Carbohydrates
PD Protein/Dairy
Ft Fats
S Sweets

Sweets

75 calories a day or 525 calories a week

Write in your calories here.

Fats

Protein/Dairy

Carbohydrates

Fruits

Vegetables

WHAT I ATE TODAY FROM THE PYRAMID:

Check off the circles in the food group servings above as you record food and beverage items in the table at left. For sweets, give your best estimate of the total number of calories for the day.

TODAY'S DATE:

TODAY'S GOAL:

NOTES ABOUT TODAY:

WHAT I ATE TODAY:

Number of servings per food group

⏱ Time	Food item	Amount	V	F	C	PD	Ft	S

GLUCOSE READINGS:

A.M. fasting	P.M. before dinner

TODAY'S ACTIVITIES:

🕐 **Time**

Total time (in minutes)	

MOTIVATION TIP:

Totally denying yourself of a food you enjoy, such as chocolate, is a sure way to fuel a craving. A more sensible approach is to treat yourself to it now and then at mealtime — but in small amounts.

KEY:

- **V** Vegetables
- **F** Fruits
- **C** Carbohydrates
- **PD** Protein/Dairy
- **Ft** Fats
- **S** Sweets

Sweets — 75 calories a day or 525 calories a week

⬅ Write in your calories here.

Fats

Protein/Dairy

Carbohydrates

Fruits

Vegetables

WHAT I ATE TODAY FROM THE PYRAMID:

Check off the circles in the food group servings above as you record food and beverage items in the table at left. For sweets, give your best estimate of the total number of calories for the day.

TODAY'S DATE:

TODAY'S GOAL:

NOTES ABOUT TODAY:

WHAT I ATE TODAY:

Number of servings per food group

🕐 Time	Food item	Amount	V	F	C	PD	Ft	S

GLUCOSE READINGS:

A.M. fasting	P.M. before dinner

TODAY'S ACTIVITIES:

	🕐 Time
Total time (in minutes)	

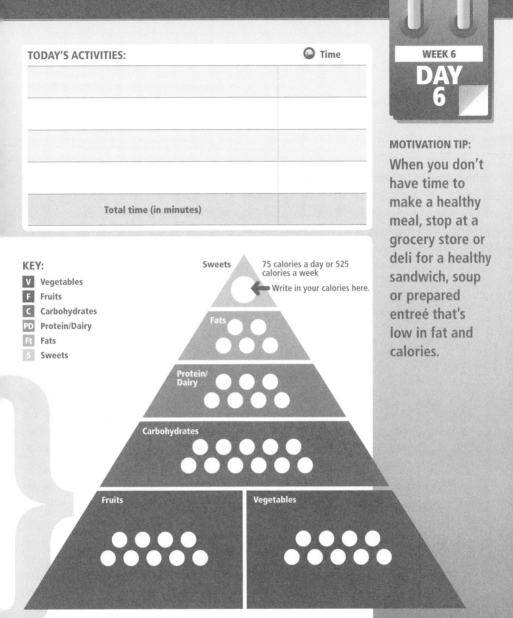

KEY:

V Vegetables
F Fruits
C Carbohydrates
PD Protein/Dairy
Ft Fats
S Sweets

Sweets
75 calories a day or 525 calories a week
← Write in your calories here.

Fats

Protein/Dairy

Carbohydrates

Fruits

Vegetables

WHAT I ATE TODAY FROM THE PYRAMID:

Check off the circles in the food group servings above as you record food and beverage items in the table at left. For sweets, give your best estimate of the total number of calories for the day.

TODAY'S DATE:

TODAY'S GOAL:

NOTES ABOUT TODAY:
It's weigh-in day ~ record my weight in the weekly Review and the Weight Record.

WHAT I ATE TODAY: Number of servings per food group

Time	Food item	Amount	V	F	C	PD	Ft	S

GLUCOSE READINGS:

A.M. fasting	P.M. before dinner

TODAY'S ACTIVITIES:

🕐 Time

Total time (in minutes)	

WEEK 6

DAY 7

REMINDER:

Record your weight for today in the weekly Review and the Weight Record.

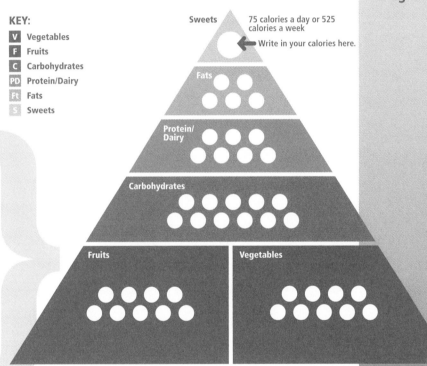

KEY:

- **V** Vegetables
- **F** Fruits
- **C** Carbohydrates
- **PD** Protein/Dairy
- **Ft** Fats
- **S** Sweets

Sweets — 75 calories a day or 525 calories a week

Write in your calories here.

Fats

Protein/Dairy

Carbohydrates

Fruits

Vegetables

WHAT I ATE TODAY FROM THE PYRAMID:

Check off the circles in the food group servings above as you record food and beverage items in the table at left. For sweets, give your best estimate of the total number of calories for the day.

My start weight ☐

Minus my weight today ☐

= Equals my weight change ☐

I FEEL:
- Terrific
- Good
- So-so
- Discouraged
- Like giving up

I'M MOST PROUD OF:

WHAT WORKED WELL:

WHAT DIDN'T WORK AS WELL:

DID I REACH MY SERVINGS GOALS FOR THIS WEEK?

Food group	Daily servings	Day 1	Day 2	Day 3	Day 4	Day 5	Day 6	Day 7
Vegetables		◯	◯	◯	◯	◯	◯	◯
Fruits		◯	◯	◯	◯	◯	◯	◯
Carbohydrates		◯	◯	◯	◯	◯	◯	◯
Protein/Dairy		◯	◯	◯	◯	◯	◯	◯
Fats		◯	◯	◯	◯	◯	◯	◯
Sweets		◯	◯	◯	◯	◯	◯	◯

DIRECTIONS:
1. Write your daily serving goals for each food group in the table above.
2. Compare the serving totals that you recorded for each day of the past week with your goals.
3. Check off the circles in the table above if your serving totals have met your goals.

CHANGES IN MY BLOOD SUGAR (GLUCOSE) READINGS:

REMINDER:
Calculate your weight change in this Review and record it in the Weight Record.

NEW FOODS OR ACTIVITIES I WOULD LIKE TO TRY:

HOW MANY STEPS A DAY DID I TAKE (IF I USED A PEDOMETER)?

Day 1	Day 2	Day 3	Day 4	Day 5	Day 6	Day 7

HOW MANY MINUTES A DAY WAS I ACTIVE?

DIRECTIONS:
1. Add a dot for your total minutes of activity for each day of last week.
2. Connect each dot on the chart with a line.

See a sample chart to the right. →

The samples above show how you can fill out your servings goals table and your activity chart for your weekly Review.

Day	Breakfast	Lunch	Dinner	Snack
EXAMPLE	cereal banana	spaghetti fruit salad	tuna wrap baby carrots	crackers and cheese
1				
2				
3				
4				
5				
6				
7				

Exercise and activities	Events and special plans
swim class @ 11am walk to work	kids ballgame @ 6pm note: supper will be on the go

WEEK AT A GLANCE

USING THE PLANNER:

Organize your plans for meals, activities and exercise in the coming week. Note upcoming events that may affect your weight program, such as travel, eating out, social occasions and vacations.

MAIN MEAL OR MEALS OF THE DAY	HOW MUCH

EASY AS 1, 2, 3:

This page allows you to check how well a meal meets your recommended servings goals.

1. Write down what you're planning to eat for this meal (or for the entire day).
2. Calculate the number of servings based on how much you're planning to eat.
3. Be sure to include the food items from your menu in your Shopping List.

PYRAMID SERVINGS FOR THIS MEAL

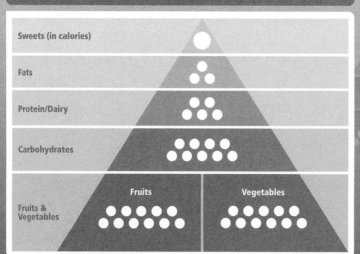

Sweets (in calories)

Fats

Protein/Dairy

Carbohydrates

Fruits &
Vegetables   Fruits   Vegetables

◄ Check off the number of servings on the pyramid at left.

MAIN MEAL OR MEALS OF THE DAY	HOW MUCH

EASY AS 1, 2, 3:

This page allows you to check how well a meal meets your recommended servings goals.

1. Write down what you're planning to eat for this meal (or for the entire day).
2. Calculate the number of servings based on how much you're planning to eat.
3. Be sure to include the food items from your menu in your Shopping List.

PYRAMID SERVINGS FOR THIS MEAL

Sweets (in calories)	○
Fats	○○○
Protein/Dairy	○○○○○
Carbohydrates	○○○○○○○○
Fruits & Vegetables	**Fruits** ○○○○○○ **Vegetables** ○○○○○○○

◄ Check off the number of servings on the pyramid at left.

MENU FOR THE DAY

BREAKFAST
1 slice whole-grain toast
1½ tbsp. jam
1 large grapefruit
Calorie-free beverage

V	F	C	PD	Ft	S
0	2	1	0	0	1

LUNCH
California Burger
1 small apple
Calorie-free beverage

V	F	C	PD	Ft	S
1	1	2	2	1	0

DINNER
1 serving Greek Salad
8 whole-grain crackers
Calorie-free beverage

V	F	C	PD	Ft	S
2	0	1	1	2	0

SNACK
*1 serving favorite vegetable
4 tbsp. fat-free sour cream

V	F	C	PD	Ft	S
1	0	0	0	1	0

*The serving size stated is the minimum amount. Eat as much as you wish.

QUICK TIP:
The menu on this page demonstrates how you can plan your own daily menus. Feel free to include this sample on one of your days.

LUNCH RECIPE

California Burger

■ Top a 3-ounce, cooked, extra-lean ground beef patty with ½ grilled onion slice, tomato slice and lettuce. Serve on a small whole-grain bun spread with 1 tablespoon low-calorie mayonnaise.

DINNER RECIPE

Greek Salad (SERVES 1)

2 C. red and green leaf lettuce
¼ C. diced cucumber
¼ C. diced sweet bell pepper
¼ C. diced carrots
¼ C. crumbled feta cheese
1 slice red onion
2 pitted Kalamata olives
2 pepperoncini peppers
1 tbsp. balsamic vinegar

■ Put lettuce in a bowl and toss with diced cucumber, bell pepper and carrots.

■ Top salad with feta cheese and onion slice, separated into rings.

■ Garnish with Kalamata olives and pepperoncini peppers.

■ Drizzle with balsamic vinegar and serve immediately.

Fresh produce	Whole grains	Meat & dairy

Frozen goods	Canned goods	Miscellaneous

QUICK TIP:

Create your shopping list for the week before going to the grocery store. You'll have all the ingredients on hand at the time you prepare a meal.

Fresh produce	Whole grains
red leaf lettuce	1 loaf whole-grain bread
green leaf lettuce	box whole-grain crackers
1 sweet bell pepper	
bag baby carrots	8 oz. package spaghetti
1 red onion	old-fashioned oatmeal
2 pepperoncini peppers	

▲
Add to your Shopping List as you plan your menus for the week.

TODAY'S DATE:

TODAY'S GOAL:

NOTES ABOUT TODAY:

WHAT I ATE TODAY: Number of servings per food group

Time	Food item	Amount	V	F	C	PD	Ft	S

GLUCOSE READINGS:

A.M. fasting	P.M. before dinner

TODAY'S ACTIVITIES:

🕐 Time

Total time (in minutes)	

MOTIVATION TIP:

To reduce stress, try organizing your day to avoid conflict and last-minute panic. Tackle unpleasant tasks early and get them over with sooner.

KEY:

- **V** Vegetables
- **F** Fruits
- **C** Carbohydrates
- **PD** Protein/Dairy
- **Ft** Fats
- **S** Sweets

Sweets

75 calories a day or 525 calories a week

← Write in your calories here.

Fats

Protein/ Dairy

Carbohydrates

Fruits

Vegetables

WHAT I ATE TODAY FROM THE PYRAMID:

Check off the circles in the food group servings above as you record food and beverage items in the table at left. For sweets, give your best estimate of the total number of calories for the day.

TODAY'S DATE:

TODAY'S GOAL:

NOTES ABOUT TODAY:

WHAT I ATE TODAY: Number of servings per food group

Time	Food item	Amount	V	F	C	PD	Ft	S

GLUCOSE READINGS:

A.M. fasting	P.M. before dinner

TODAY'S ACTIVITIES:

🕐 **Time**

Total time (in minutes)	

WEEK 7

DAY
2

MOTIVATION TIP:

To cut down on snacking at the movie theater, eat something healthy before you leave home. Drink water or a calorie-free beverage while you're there.

KEY:

V	Vegetables
F	Fruits
C	Carbohydrates
PD	Protein/Dairy
Ft	Fats
S	Sweets

Sweets

75 calories a day or 525 calories a week

← Write in your calories here.

Fats

Protein/ Dairy

Carbohydrates

Fruits

Vegetables

WHAT I ATE TODAY FROM THE PYRAMID:

Check off the circles in the food group servings above as you record food and beverage items in the table at left. For sweets, give your best estimate of the total number of calories for the day.

TODAY'S DATE:

TODAY'S GOAL:

NOTES ABOUT TODAY:

WHAT I ATE TODAY: **Number of servings per food group**

⏱ Time	Food item	Amount	V	F	C	PD	Ft	S

GLUCOSE READINGS:

A.M. fasting	P.M. before dinner

TODAY'S ACTIVITIES:

	Time
Total time (in minutes)	

MOTIVATION TIP:
Mix things up when you exercise. Don't feel tied to just one type of activity, such as walking. Occasionally, try biking or swimming instead.

KEY:
- **V** Vegetables
- **F** Fruits
- **C** Carbohydrates
- **PD** Protein/Dairy
- **Ft** Fats
- **S** Sweets

Sweets — 75 calories a day or 525 calories a week

Write in your calories here.

Fats

Protein/Dairy

Carbohydrates

Fruits

Vegetables

WHAT I ATE TODAY FROM THE PYRAMID:
Check off the circles in the food group servings above as you record food and beverage items in the table at left. For sweets, give your best estimate of the total number of calories for the day.

TODAY'S DATE:

TODAY'S GOAL:

NOTES ABOUT TODAY:

WHAT I ATE TODAY: Number of servings per food group

Time	Food item	Amount	V	F	C	PD	Ft	S

GLUCOSE READINGS:

A.M. fasting	P.M. before dinner

TODAY'S ACTIVITIES:

⏱ Time

Total time (in minutes)	

MOTIVATION TIP:
Consider growing some of your own produce. It's not as hard as you may think. If you don't have space for a garden plot, you can grow items such as tomatoes and peppers in outdoor pots.

KEY:
- **V** Vegetables
- **F** Fruits
- **C** Carbohydrates
- **PD** Protein/Dairy
- **Ft** Fats
- **S** Sweets

Sweets — 75 calories a day or 525 calories a week
← Write in your calories here.

Fats

Protein/Dairy

Carbohydrates

Fruits   Vegetables

WHAT I ATE TODAY FROM THE PYRAMID:

Check off the circles in the food group servings above as you record food and beverage items in the table at left. For sweets, give your best estimate of the total number of calories for the day.

TODAY'S DATE:

TODAY'S GOAL:

NOTES ABOUT TODAY:

WHAT I ATE TODAY:

Number of servings per food group

⏱ Time	Food item	Amount	V	F	C	PD	Ft	S

GLUCOSE READINGS:

A.M. fasting	P.M. before dinner

TODAY'S ACTIVITIES:

	⏱ Time
Total time (in minutes)	

MOTIVATION TIP:
Counteract all-or-nothing thinking. Try not to label a food as being either "good" or "bad." You can eat most foods in moderation. It's even OK to have dessert once in a while.

KEY:

- **V** Vegetables
- **F** Fruits
- **C** Carbohydrates
- **PD** Protein/Dairy
- **Ft** Fats
- **S** Sweets

Sweets — 75 calories a day or 525 calories a week
← Write in your calories here.

Fats

Protein/Dairy

Carbohydrates

Fruits

Vegetables

WHAT I ATE TODAY FROM THE PYRAMID:
Check off the circles in the food group servings above as you record food and beverage items in the table at left. For sweets, give your best estimate of the total number of calories for the day.

TODAY'S DATE:

TODAY'S GOAL:

NOTES ABOUT TODAY:

WHAT I ATE TODAY: Number of servings per food group

⏱ Time	Food item	Amount	V	F	C	PD	Ft	S

GLUCOSE READINGS:

A.M. fasting	P.M. before dinner

TODAY'S ACTIVITIES:

	⏱ Time
Total time (in minutes)	

WEEK 7
DAY
6

MOTIVATION TIP:

Try to build your self-esteem. Don't hide behind oversized, drab clothing. Dress in clothing that makes you feel good about yourself.

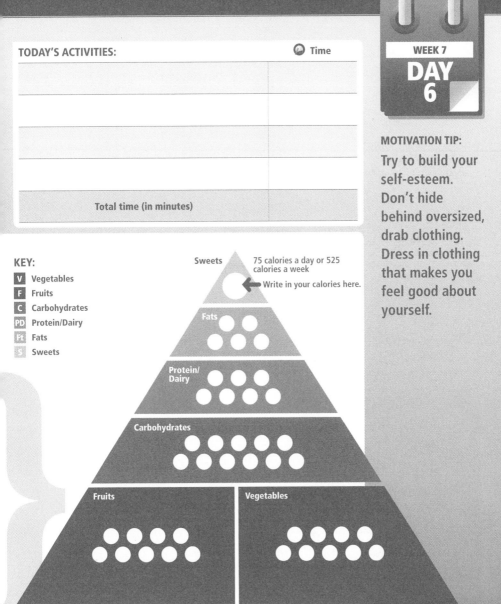

KEY:
- **V** Vegetables
- **F** Fruits
- **C** Carbohydrates
- **PD** Protein/Dairy
- **Ft** Fats
- **S** Sweets

Sweets — 75 calories a day or 525 calories a week
Write in your calories here.

Fats

Protein/Dairy

Carbohydrates

Fruits

Vegetables

WHAT I ATE TODAY FROM THE PYRAMID:

Check off the circles in the food group servings above as you record food and beverage items in the table at left. For sweets, give your best estimate of the total number of calories for the day.

TODAY'S DATE:

TODAY'S GOAL:

NOTES ABOUT TODAY:
It's weigh-in day ~ record my weight in the weekly Review and the Weight Record.

WHAT I ATE TODAY: Number of servings per food group

⏱ Time	Food item	Amount	V	F	C	PD	Ft	S

GLUCOSE READINGS:

A.M. fasting	P.M. before dinner

TODAY'S ACTIVITIES:

	⏱ Time
Total time (in minutes)	

REMINDER: 🔲
Record your weight for today in the weekly Review and the Weight Record.

KEY:
- **V** Vegetables
- **F** Fruits
- **C** Carbohydrates
- **PD** Protein/Dairy
- **Ft** Fats
- **S** Sweets

Sweets — 75 calories a day or 525 calories a week
← Write in your calories here.

Fats

Protein/Dairy

Carbohydrates

Fruits

Vegetables

WHAT I ATE TODAY FROM THE PYRAMID:

Check off the circles in the food group servings above as you record food and beverage items in the table at left. For sweets, give your best estimate of the total number of calories for the day.

My start weight	
Minus my weight today	
= Equals my weight change	

I FEEL:
- Terrific
- Good
- So-so
- Discouraged
- Like giving up

I'M MOST PROUD OF:

WHAT WORKED WELL:

WHAT DIDN'T WORK AS WELL:

DID I REACH MY SERVINGS GOALS FOR THIS WEEK?

Food group	Daily servings	Day 1	Day 2	Day 3	Day 4	Day 5	Day 6	Day 7
Vegetables		○	○	○	○	○	○	○
Fruits		○	○	○	○	○	○	○
Carbohydrates		○	○	○	○	○	○	○
Protein/Dairy		○	○	○	○	○	○	○
Fats		○	○	○	○	○	○	○
Sweets		○	○	○	○	○	○	○

DIRECTIONS:
1. Write your daily serving goals for each food group in the table above.
2. Compare the serving totals that you recorded for each day of the past week with your goals.
3. Check off the circles in the table above if your serving totals have met your goals.

CHANGES IN MY BLOOD SUGAR (GLUCOSE) READINGS:

NEW FOODS OR ACTIVITIES I WOULD LIKE TO TRY:

HOW MANY STEPS A DAY DID I TAKE (IF I USED A PEDOMETER)?

Day 1	Day 2	Day 3	Day 4	Day 5	Day 6	Day 7

REMINDER: Calculate your weight change in this Review and record it in the Weight Record.

HOW MANY MINUTES A DAY WAS I ACTIVE?

DIRECTIONS:

1. Add a dot for your total minutes of activity for each day of last week.
2. Connect each dot on the chart with a line.

See a sample chart to the right. →

The samples above show how you can fill out your servings goals table and your activity chart for your weekly Review.

Day	Breakfast	Lunch	Dinner	Snack
EXAMPLE	cereal banana	spaghetti fruit salad	tuna wrap baby carrots	crackers and cheese
1				
2				
3				
4				
5				
6				
7				

Exercise and activities	Events and special plans
swim class @ 11am walk to work	kids ballgame @ 6pm note: supper will be on the go

USING THE PLANNER:

Organize your plans for meals, activities and exercise in the coming week. Note upcoming events that may affect your weight program, such as travel, eating out, social occasions and vacations.

MEAL PLANNER

MAIN MEAL OR MEALS OF THE DAY	HOW MUCH

EASY AS 1, 2, 3:

This page allows you to check how well a meal meets your recommended servings goals.

1. Write down what you're planning to eat for this meal (or for the entire day).

2. Calculate the number of servings based on how much you're planning to eat.

3. Be sure to include the food items from your menu in your Shopping List.

PYRAMID SERVINGS FOR THIS MEAL

Sweets (in calories)	●
Fats	●● ●
Protein/Dairy	●●● ●●
Carbohydrates	●●●● ●●●●
Fruits & Vegetables	**Fruits** ●●●●● ●●●●● **Vegetables** ●●●●● ●●●●●

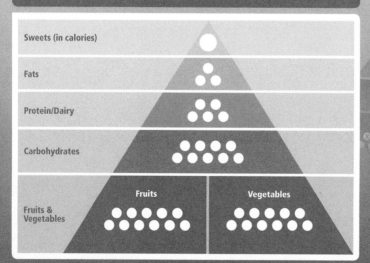

◀ Check off the number of servings on the pyramid at left.

MAIN MEAL OR MEALS OF THE DAY	HOW MUCH

EASY AS 1, 2, 3:

This page allows you to check how well a meal meets your recommended servings goals.

1. Write down what you're planning to eat for this meal (or for the entire day).

2. Calculate the number of servings based on how much you're planning to eat.

3. Be sure to include the food items from your menu in your Shopping List.

PYRAMID SERVINGS FOR THIS MEAL

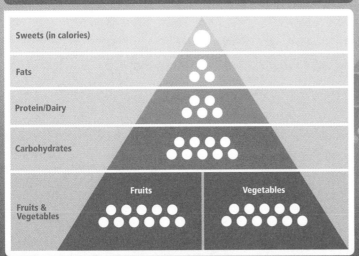

Sweets (in calories)	○
Fats	
Protein/Dairy	
Carbohydrates	
Fruits & Vegetables	Fruits / Vegetables

75

◄ Check off the number of servings on the pyramid at left.

MENU FOR THE DAY

BREAKFAST
Breakfast Burrito
1 medium orange
Calorie-free beverage

V	F	C	PD	Ft	S
1	1	2	1	0	0

LUNCH
Spinach Fruit Salad
2 tbsp. fat-free French dressing
1 c. skim milk
8 whole peanuts or 4 whole cashews
Calorie-free beverage

V	F	C	PD	Ft	S
2	1	0	1	2	0

DINNER
3 oz. fish or shrimp, broiled or grilled
⅔ c. cooked brown rice
*1 c. steamed broccoli
*2 c. lettuce
2 tbsp. fat-free salad dressing
1 c. mixed berries
Calorie-free beverage

V	F	C	PD	Ft	S
2	1	2	1	1	0

SNACK
1 serving favorite fruit

V	F	C	PD	Ft	S
0	1	0	0	0	0

*The serving size stated is the minimum amount. Eat as much as you wish.

QUICK TIP:

The menu on this page demonstrates how you can plan your own daily menus. Feel free to include this sample on one of your days.

BREAKFAST RECIPE

Breakfast Burrito

■ Sauté ½ cup chopped tomato, 2 tablespoons chopped onion and ¼ cup canned corn with some of its liquid. Add ½ cup egg substitute and scramble with vegetables. Spread on a fat-free tortilla, roll up the tortilla, and top with 2 tablespoons of salsa.

LUNCH RECIPE

Spinach Fruit Salad

■ Top 2 cups of baby spinach with ½ cup green pepper strips and water chestnuts, and ½ cup mandarin orange sections.

Fresh produce	Whole grains	Meat & dairy

Frozen goods	Canned goods	Miscellaneous

QUICK TIP:

Create your shopping list for the week before going to the grocery store. You'll have all the ingredients on hand at the time you prepare a meal.

Fresh produce	Whole grains
1 medium tomato	whole-wheat tortillas
1 bunch green onions	brown rice
mushrooms	1 package English muffin
1 green onion	box whole-gra crackers
spinach	
lettuce	
broccoli	

Add to your Shopping List as you plan your menus for the week.

TODAY'S DATE:

TODAY'S GOAL:

NOTES ABOUT TODAY:

WHAT I ATE TODAY: Number of servings per food group

🕐 Time	Food item	Amount	V	F	C	PD	Ft	S

GLUCOSE READINGS:

A.M. fasting	P.M. before dinner

TODAY'S ACTIVITIES:

🕐 **Time**

Total time (in minutes)	

MOTIVATION TIP:

If you can stay focused on a healthy lifestyle, the weight will take care of itself. That includes a balanced diet, daily physical activity, getting enough sleep and managing stress.

KEY:

- **V** Vegetables
- **F** Fruits
- **C** Carbohydrates
- **PD** Protein/Dairy
- **Ft** Fats
- **S** Sweets

Sweets — 75 calories a day or 525 calories a week
← Write in your calories here.

Fats

Protein/Dairy

Carbohydrates

Fruits

Vegetables

WHAT I ATE TODAY FROM THE PYRAMID:

Check off the circles in the food group servings above as you record food and beverage items in the table at left. For sweets, give your best estimate of the total number of calories for the day.

TODAY'S DATE:

TODAY'S GOAL:

NOTES ABOUT TODAY:

WHAT I ATE TODAY:　　　　　　　　　　　Number of servings per food group

🕐 Time	Food item	Amount	V	F	C	PD	Ft	S

GLUCOSE READINGS:

A.M. fasting	P.M. before dinner

TODAY'S ACTIVITIES:

	⏱ Time
Total time (in minutes)	

MOTIVATION TIP:
To continue losing weight or maintaining the weight you have, keep doing whatever worked for you in the past. You can always adapt tried-and-true strategies to meet changing circumstances.

KEY:

V Vegetables
F Fruits
C Carbohydrates
PD Protein/Dairy
Ft Fats
S Sweets

Sweets — 75 calories a day or 525 calories a week
Write in your calories here.

Fats

Protein/Dairy

Carbohydrates

Fruits

Vegetables

WHAT I ATE TODAY FROM THE PYRAMID:
Check off the circles in the food group servings above as you record food and beverage items in the table at left. For sweets, give your best estimate of the total number of calories for the day.

TODAY'S DATE:

TODAY'S GOAL:

NOTES ABOUT TODAY:

WHAT I ATE TODAY: Number of servings per food group

🕐 Time	Food item	Amount	V	F	C	PD	Ft	S

GLUCOSE READINGS:

A.M. fasting	P.M. before dinner

TODAY'S ACTIVITIES:

	🕐 **Time**
Total time (in minutes)	

MOTIVATION TIP:
What you do to maintain your weight should be things you look forward to doing. You want to make weight control enjoyable and comforting, not unpleasant and tiresome.

KEY:

V	Vegetables
F	Fruits
C	Carbohydrates
PD	Protein/Dairy
Ft	Fats
S	Sweets

Sweets — 75 calories a day or 525 calories a week
→ Write in your calories here.

Fats

Protein/Dairy

Carbohydrates

Fruits

Vegetables

WHAT I ATE TODAY FROM THE PYRAMID:
Check off the circles in the food group servings above as you record food and beverage items in the table at left. For sweets, give your best estimate of the total number of calories for the day.

TODAY'S DATE:

TODAY'S GOAL:

NOTES ABOUT TODAY:

WHAT I ATE TODAY: Number of servings per food group

⏱ Time	Food item	Amount	V	F	C	PD	Ft	S

GLUCOSE READINGS:

A.M. fasting	P.M. before dinner

TODAY'S ACTIVITIES:

	⏱ Time
Total time (in minutes)	

MOTIVATION TIP:

Regardless of how much weight you've lost, the fact that you've stayed with the program and continued to use the journal for this long is an important achievement.

KEY:

V Vegetables
F Fruits
C Carbohydrates
PD Protein/Dairy
Ft Fats
S Sweets

Sweets   75 calories a day or 525 calories a week
← Write in your calories here.

Fats

Protein/Dairy

Carbohydrates

Fruits   Vegetables

WHAT I ATE TODAY FROM THE PYRAMID:

Check off the circles in the food group servings above as you record food and beverage items in the table at left. For sweets, give your best estimate of the total number of calories for the day.

TODAY'S DATE:

TODAY'S GOAL:

NOTES ABOUT TODAY:

WHAT I ATE TODAY: Number of servings per food group

🕐 Time	Food item	Amount	V	F	C	PD	Ft	S

GLUCOSE READINGS:

A.M. fasting	P.M. before dinner

TODAY'S ACTIVITIES: 🕐 **Time**

Total time (in minutes)	

KEY:

V	Vegetables
F	Fruits
C	Carbohydrates
PD	Protein/Dairy
Ft	Fats
S	Sweets

Sweets — 75 calories a day or 525 calories a week

← Write in your calories here.

Fats

Protein/ Dairy

Carbohydrates

Fruits   **Vegetables**

MOTIVATION TIP:

Make a list of the people you most admire. This may include parents, children, educators, scientists and world leaders. Do they have perfect bodies? Does it really matter?

WHAT I ATE TODAY FROM THE PYRAMID:

Check off the circles in the food group servings above as you record food and beverage items in the table at left. For sweets, give your best estimate of the total number of calories for the day.

TODAY'S DATE:

TODAY'S GOAL:

NOTES ABOUT TODAY:

WHAT I ATE TODAY: Number of servings per food group

⏱ Time	Food item	Amount	V	F	C	PD	Ft	S

GLUCOSE READINGS:

A.M. fasting	P.M. before dinner

TODAY'S ACTIVITIES:

⏱ Time

Total time (in minutes)	

MOTIVATION TIP:
Doing something nice for someone else can boost your self-esteem. Send a card or flowers to someone, offer assistance or do volunteer work in your community.

KEY:

V	Vegetables
F	Fruits
C	Carbohydrates
PD	Protein/Dairy
Ft	Fats
S	Sweets

Sweets

75 calories a day or 525 calories a week

← Write in your calories here.

Fats

Protein/Dairy

Carbohydrates

Fruits

Vegetables

WHAT I ATE TODAY FROM THE PYRAMID:
Check off the circles in the food group servings above as you record food and beverage items in the table at left. For sweets, give your best estimate of the total number of calories for the day.

TODAY'S DATE:

TODAY'S GOAL:

NOTES ABOUT TODAY:
It's weigh-in day ~ record my weight in the weekly Review and the Weight Record.

WHAT I ATE TODAY:

Number of servings per food group

⏱ Time	Food item	Amount	V	F	C	PD	Ft	S

GLUCOSE READINGS:

A.M. fasting	P.M. before dinner

TODAY'S ACTIVITIES:

⏱ Time

Total time (in minutes)	

REMINDER:

Record your weight for today in the weekly Review and the Weight Record.

KEY:

V	Vegetables
F	Fruits
C	Carbohydrates
PD	Protein/Dairy
Ft	Fats
S	Sweets

Sweets

75 calories a day or 525 calories a week

← Write in your calories here.

Fats

Protein/Dairy

Carbohydrates

Fruits

Vegetables

WHAT I ATE TODAY FROM THE PYRAMID:

Check off the circles in the food group servings above as you record food and beverage items in the table at left. For sweets, give your best estimate of the total number of calories for the day.

My start weight [_____]

Minus my weight today [_____]

= Equals my weight change [_____]

I FEEL:
- Terrific
- Good
- So-so
- Discouraged
- Like giving up

I'M MOST PROUD OF:

WHAT WORKED WELL:

WHAT DIDN'T WORK AS WELL:

DID I REACH MY SERVINGS GOALS FOR THIS WEEK?

Food group	Daily servings	Day 1	Day 2	Day 3	Day 4	Day 5	Day 6	Day 7
Vegetables		○	○	○	○	○	○	○
Fruits		○	○	○	○	○	○	○
Carbohydrates		○	○	○	○	○	○	○
Protein/Dairy		○	○	○	○	○	○	○
Fats		○	○	○	○	○	○	○
Sweets		○	○	○	○	○	○	○

DIRECTIONS:
1. Write your daily serving goals for each food group in the table above.
2. Compare the serving totals that you recorded for each day of the past week with your goals.
3. Check off the circles in the table above if your serving totals have met your goals.

CHANGES IN MY BLOOD SUGAR (GLUCOSE) READINGS:

NEW FOODS OR ACTIVITIES I WOULD LIKE TO TRY:

HOW MANY STEPS A DAY DID I TAKE (IF I USED A PEDOMETER)?

Day 1	Day 2	Day 3	Day 4	Day 5	Day 6	Day 7

HOW MANY MINUTES A DAY WAS I ACTIVE?

Days

(Activity chart: Minutes axis marked 0, 15, 30, 45, 60, 75, 90; Days axis marked 1, 2, 3, 4, 5, 6, 7)

DIRECTIONS:
1. Add a dot for your total minutes of activity for each day of last week.
2. Connect each dot on the chart with a line.

See a sample chart to the right. →

REMINDER:
It's time to have an A1C test again to see if your results have improved (see page 7). Ask your doctor for the test and record the results in the box on this page.

DID I REACH MY SERVINGS GOALS FOR THIS

Food group	Daily servings	Day 1	D
Vegetables	4+	✓	
Fruits	3+		
Carbohydrates	4	✓	
Protein/Dairy	3	✓	✓
Fats	3		✓

The samples above show how you can fill out your servings goals table and your activity chart for your weekly Review.

Making healthy weight a lifetime commitment

Think about the goals you set for yourself at the start of *The Mayo Clinic Diabetes Diet*. Ten weeks later, do the results meet your expectations?

Judging your progress strictly in terms of the numbers — your weight when you started compared to your weight now — may satisfy you or you may end up feeling disappointed. Many people believe they can never lose enough weight, producing an endless cycle of "dieting."

Weight control isn't only about the number of pounds you lose. Consider how your efforts have equipped you to better control your diabetes — or perhaps even prevented you from developing diabetes.

Don't forget that because of your efforts, you're now eating better and you're more active. Think about the new strategies you've learned to help overcome obstacles and change unhealthy behaviors. Recall all the foods and recipes you've sampled and enjoyed. All of these changes have combined to make you healthier.

Any amount of weight you've lost, no matter how small, is a step toward a healthier you. At this time, if you feel that you need to lose more weight, you can continue doing what you've been doing. If you're satisfied with the weight you've lost, then your attention turns to keeping those pounds off.

Strategies for a lifetime

Regardless of which path you choose to take — losing more weight or staying at the weight you're at — *The Mayo Clinic Diabetes Diet* has given you the resources you'll need to achieve your weight goal.

Here are basic guidelines that may help you incorporate what you've learned into a lifetime of healthy living:

Stick to the basics

Continue to focus on maintaining a healthy lifestyle, and the weight will take care of itself. Stick to a balanced diet, moderate portions and daily physical activity. Get enough sleep and try to manage stress. Remember that these factors are something that everyone should strive to do in life, not just individuals who are intent on losing weight.

Persistence pays off

Keep doing whatever worked for you in the past. Adapt these strategies to new situations. Vary or add to them to make your program more stimulating or challenging.

Your ultimate goal is to incorporate the new, healthy behaviors that you've learned in the diet into your daily life. You don't want to set them aside after 10 weeks and revert back to your old ways of doing things.

Make it enjoyable

The things you do to maintain your weight should be things that you look forward to doing. You want them to be enjoyable and comforting, not unpleasant and tiresome. As soon as you start finding excuses or dragging your feet, these new behaviors will be quickly cast aside.

Keep a long-term perspective

Regardless of how many pounds you may have lost, the fact that you've stayed with the program may be your most important achievement.

It's important to consider weight control beyond a 10-week or 10-month or even 10-year period. It's for a lifetime. And no matter what your expectations may be, by staying committed, you'll reach your goal — perhaps sooner than you think.

Give yourself credit

Acknowledge the vital role you've played in making your program a success. It was your commitment to losing weight that got you started. It was your energy and persistence that kept you going. You should now have the tools and experience to continue on. Giving yourself credit for what you've accomplished helps raise your confidence level so that you can manage whatever challenges may come along in the future.

Looking forward

In the months and years ahead, take time occasionally to reconfirm your commitment to maintaining a healthy weight and managing your blood sugar (glucose). Remind yourself of the many benefits you receive from a healthy lifestyle.

Don't ignore negative feelings or emotions that you may have regarding your efforts — try to determine their causes and look for solutions. Over time, adapt your program or include different strategies in light of changing needs and circumstances.

You've used weigh-ins throughout the 10 weeks of *The Mayo Clinic Diabetes Diet Journal* to track your progress and keep you motivated. You might find it helpful to continue keeping weight and blood sugar records, even if you've completed the journal.

WEEK 1 HABIT TRACKER								
✓ Check if done	Day 1	Day 2	Day 3	Day 4	Day 5	Day 6	Day 7	TOTALS
ADD 5 HABITS								
1. Eat a healthy breakfast								
2. Eat vegetables and fruits								
3. Eat whole grains								
4. Eat healthy fats								
5. Move!								
BREAK 5 HABITS								
1. No TV while eating								
2. No sugar								
3. No snacks								
4. Only moderate meat and dairy								
5. No eating at restaurants								
5 BONUS HABITS								
1. Keep diet records								
2. Keep exercise/activity records								
3. Move more!								
4. Eat "real" food								
5. Write your daily goals								
Totals								

DIRECTIONS:

1. At the end of each day, check off which Add, Break and Bonus habits you have completed.
2. At the end of the week, total the columns and the rows to see how you've progressed.

WEEK 2 HABIT TRACKER							
Day 8	Day 9	Day 10	Day 11	Day 12	Day 13	Day 14	TOTALS
ADD 5 HABITS							
BREAK 5 HABITS							
5 BONUS HABITS							

REMINDER:

Total the columns and rows of your Habit Tracker to see which habits you're having success with and which are a problem for you.

See pages 66-67 of The Mayo Clinic Diabetes Diet.

WEEK 1 HABIT TRA			
✓ Check if done	Day 1	Day 2	Day 3
ADD 5 HABITS			
1. Eat a healthy breakfast	✓	✓	
2. Eat vegetables and fruits	✓	✓	✓
3. Eat whole grains	✓	✓	✓
4. Eat healthy fats	✓	✓	✓
5. Move!	✓		✓
BREAK 5 HABITS			
1. No TV while eating			
2. No sugar	✓	✓	
3. No snacks	✓	✓	
4. Only moderate meat and dairy	✓	✓	
5. No eating at restaurants	✓	✓	
5 BONUS HABITS			
1. Keep diet records		✓	

The sample above demonstrates how to fill out your Habit Tracker.

Lose It!

DAILY RECORD · **DAY** ☐

TODAY'S DATE

TODAY'S GOAL:

TODAY'S ACTIVITIES:

	🕐 Time
Total time (in minutes)	

REMINDER: 🔔
Remember to weigh yourself at the end of each week.

WHAT I ATE TODAY:

🕐 Time	Food item	Amount

GLUCOSE READINGS:

A.M. fasting	P.M. before dinner

Lose It!

DAILY RECORD · DAY

TODAY'S GOAL:

TODAY'S ACTIVITIES: ⏱ Time

Total time (in minutes)	

TODAY'S DATE

REMINDER:
Remember to weigh yourself at the end of each week.

WHAT I ATE TODAY:

⏱ Time	Food item	Amount

GLUCOSE READINGS:

A.M. fasting	P.M. before dinner

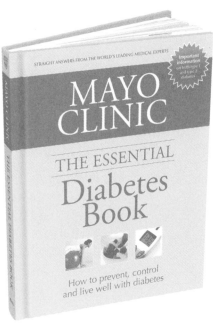

Take Control of Your Health ...

In *Mayo Clinic The Essential Diabetes Book,* you'll find the latest guidelines on diagnosis and testing, as well as valuable self-care tips. You'll learn the best ways we know to prevent or manage diabetes, and why i is so vital to reduce your risk.

**This book has the latest help
Mayo Clinic can offer so you can live better with diabetes.**

- Why is diabetes so prevalent today — have our genes changed? The answer is no, but other things have ... and the good news is that you have control over those "other things."

- Are you at risk of developing type 2 diabetes? Our eight-point checklist reveals the answer.

- Whether your risk is high or low, knowing the seven signs and symptoms of diabetes is vital to getting appropriate treatment much more quickly.

- For some people, lifestyle changes aren't enough and medications are necessary to maintain healthy blood sugar levels. Find comprehensive coverage on insulin therapy, various insulin options, oral medications for type 2 diabetes, oral drug combinations, new drug approaches and some experimental procedures now being researched.

- Diabetes can't be cured, but it may be prevented — if you take the right steps. And if you already have diabetes, the treatments are better than ever.

I decided to go to Mayo Clinic. It was like nothing I'd ever seen before. The doctors are true specialists and the personal care is amazing. I wish that I'd gone there first. My answer was Mayo Clinic.

MICHELLE FRITS
Lake in the Hills, Illinois

For more than 100 years, people from all walks of life have found answers at Mayo Clinic. We work with many insurance companies and are an in-network provider for millions of people. To make an appointment, please visit *www.MayoClinic.org*. In most cases, a physician referral is not needed.

SCOTTSDALE, ROCHESTER, JACKSONVILLE,
ARIZONA MINNESOTA FLORIDA

MAYO CLINIC

Three Wonderful Companions!

For stove-top and oven cooking—

By *New York Times* bestselling author Phyllis Pellman Good with the American Diabetes Association

These cookbooks make mealtime an occasion when everyone belongs!

For slow-cooker recipes—

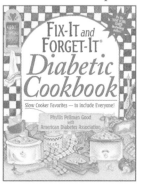

Fix-It and Enjoy-It Diabetic Cookbook (520 great recipes)

Fix-It and Forget-It Diabetic Cookbook (600 great recipes)

Published in cooperation with

American Diabetes Association

Cure • Care • Commitment®

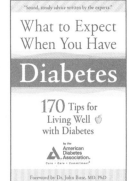

What to Expect When You Have Diabetes is sound, steadying advice written by the experts, so you can live well with diabetes, not just manage it.

A Q&A format, in straightforward language and organized by topic for quick reference, makes this **a perfect companion to a health-care team**.

What to Expect When You Have Diabetes: 170 Tips for Living Well with Diabetes